Live Better While You Age

Live Better While You Age

Tips and Tools for a Healthier, Longer Life

James W. Jones

ROWMAN & LITTLEFIELD
Lanham • Boulder • New York • London

This book represents reference material only. It is not intended as a medical manual, and the data presented here are meant to assist the reader in making informed choices. This book is not a replacement for treatment(s) that the reader's personal physician may have suggested. If the reader believes he or she is experiencing a medical issue, professional medical help is recommended. Mention of particular products, companies, or authorities in this book does not indicate endorsement by the publisher or author.

Published by Rowman & Littlefield
A wholly owned subsidary of The Rowman & Littlefield Publishing Group, Inc.
4501 Forbes Boulevard, Suite 200, Lanham, Maryland 20706
www.rowman.com

Unit A, Whitacre Mews, 26-34 Stannary Street, London SE11 4AB

British Library Cataloguing in Publication Information Available

Library of Congress Cataloging-in-Publication Data
Names: Jones, James W. (James Wilson), 1941- author.
Title: Live better while you age : tips and tools for a healthier, longer life / James W. Jones.
Description: Lanham : Rowman & Littlefield, [2016] | Includes bibliographical references and index.
Identifiers: LCCN 2016028527 (print) | LCCN 2016037458 (ebook) | ISBN 9781442269583 (cloth : alk. paper) | ISBN 9781442269590 (electronic)
Subjects: LCSH: Self-care, Health—Popular works. | Aging—Prevention—Popular works.
Classification: LCC RA776.95 .J65 2016 (print) | LCC RA776.95 (ebook) | DDC 613.2—dc23
LC record available at https://lccn.loc.gov/2016028527

∞™ The paper used in this publication meets the minimum requirements of American National Standard for Information Sciences—Permanence of Paper for Printed Library Materials, ANSI/NISO Z39.48-1992.

Printed in the United States of America

This book is dedicated to Mary Nichols, my grandmother, who was a nurse and the most caring person I have known. She never learned to drive a car so she would walk miles to do chores, such as shopping.
Her entire backyard was a garden with fruit trees and she loved their yields. She canned enough to last all year. She lived to be a hundred and one and was independent until the last making quilts which she sold.

Contents

PART III: MEDICAL CARE AND MANAGEMENT 137

Introduction

Just like books on "how to make a million," there are many health and wellness books. The more instructional ways that exist on a subject, the less the chance of finding the perfect answer. Also, many books advising healthy habits feel they need to wow people with "man bites dog" stories, which are misleading at best. I believe that offering practical evidence-based information as clearly as possible is the best instructional method.

The best approach to a complex question is to examine the topic's foundational issues wherein lies the answer. Eye-opening answers professors bestow in medical school are called pearls. "Clinical pearls are best defined as small bits of free standing, clinically relevant information based on experience or observation."[1] I want to achieve many "why didn't I think of that" moments for the reader.

Obviously, reasonable people want to enjoy robust lives, free from the ravages of aging and aging-related diseases. The question is how to secure that admirable goal. Numerous books address preserving health but none is comprehensive and approaches successful aging from a scientific methodology. Invariably, piecemeal efforts to describe aspects of attaining health include fitness, emotional aspects, or, most commonly, diet, and they offer authoritative opinions. Be aware, there is a huge difference between knowledge and opinion. Opinion is without data; it is arguable and different "authorities" disagree. Do not base your health program on opinion; it is gambling with your future—big time. The last decade exploded with scientific data about aging successfully. Throughout this book, I have collected and triply distilled the wisdom that data holds. Middle-aged people don't think much about maintaining their health because they have not noticed declines. Declines will come. I can no longer bench press 250 pounds but I don't need or want to do so. The objective should be to limit declines so the quality of life remains good and you can do what you want to do. Nevertheless, the sooner one chooses a constructive lifestyle, the more benefits they gain. Measurable benefits are attainable even when changes are made in one's 70s.

This book's purpose is to provide the reader with a primer that includes principles necessary for living a better life. I believe in the foundation of knowledge attributed to, but described before the philosopher Spinoza—The Principle of Sufficient Reason. It states simply that everything that happens has a reason for happening. Amazingly, we generally apply that wisdom to everything in our lives, except our bodies.

Professor Haidt and others propose that contrary to our beliefs the majority of our choices, especially about behaviors, are decided by our unconscious mind. Haidt compares the interaction to a person (conscious mind) riding an elephant (unconscious mind).[2] Our consciousness thinks we are in charge but we are often in an advisory role. Moreover, our health is the result of our behaviors—mostly chosen by our elephant, unless we train the elephant. This book tells you how to train your elephant.

The book attempts to bring you the essence of 16 of the most important areas regarding your healthful living by presenting the most important data proven wisdom. Prevention of biological corrosion is important but is just one area of better, more rewarding living that we will explore.

Almost everything important having to do with our well-being is incremental with increments that are incredibly minute. Seven out of ten deaths in America are incrementally acquired and over 90% are avoidable by choices. The incremental diseases are termed "chronic" when a better term is "aging-related," or even better "lifestyle-related." The non-lifestyle-related causes of death (and disability) that mostly are avoidable are suicide and some injuries.

The approach I embrace is not to concentrate on health-promoting lifestyle behaviors but to concentrate on the reasons why certain behaviors are beneficial or harmful. With scientific evidence–based facts, one can design their personal, best lifestyle approach. Readers should not be automatons following a specific program; instead, they need to understand the underpinnings of successful aging and then they will know how to mature successfully.

Part I

THE AGING BODY

Chapter 1

Motivation Inspiration

Stop, Breathe, Think, Then Act

In my late thirties, I took up scuba diving. I'd always wanted to experience the sensation of being nearly weightless underwater, gliding along, breathing naturally, and observing marine life up close. I'm sure I've forgotten much of what the then-young instructor had told us about how to defog a mask or properly clean a wet suit. But what I will never forget is what he said that first day—and this was before we even got wet. "Divers!" he barked. "Obey the rules or death is minutes away."

That stuck with me. He went on, his voice an octave higher, making sure he had all of us with him. "If there is anything to remember it is this: Stop! Breathe! Think! Then act. It is the most important rule in scuba diving. It one day might save your life."

Good health is largely achievable by following the same advice. (And, just like diving, ignoring the rules brings about your demise much sooner.) Following the rules saved my life when diving. When in Palau (a group of isolated islands in the South Pacific), I went diving in a multi-chambered cave named the Chandelier. My guide and I went into the cave, as a group of inexperienced divers exited. They stirred the sediment, a real no-no in cave diving, so visibility became so bad that I lost track of my guide who kept swimming onward. Soon I could no longer hear my guide; I was alone in the darkness. I stopped, took a deep breath, thought, and then acted. Otherwise, I would suck my tank empty of air and die. I noted the guide was very experienced diving this cave, so he must have swum directly to an opening in the chamber that led to the outside. I noted the reading of my depth gage and angle of ascent and kept to the same route. To proceed otherwise may have

3

taken me into a wrong chamber. I surfaced in the correct chamber, took off my mask, and the local guide blurted, "where you beeeen?"

Danger is so apparent in scuba diving; death's bony finger is clearly visible. Death's bony finger is just as clear in our unhealthy lifestyles but we often choose to ignore warnings. We must be in denial. We consider ourselves exempt from the statistics declaring that if you embrace unhealthy behaviors, you will suffer. Denial is a well-developed human trait. I was billeted at a Marine Corps base during the Vietnam War during which 58,220 ill-fated soldiers who thought they were invincible died. No one is invincible.

What on Earth makes you think the health statistics don't apply to you? Proven threats apply to us all equally. It obviously does, but why should it matter whether the actual dying takes a few minutes or several decades? Remember, also, suffering in one instance is a few minutes, compared possibly suffering for months in the other. Without healthy living, one is slowly drowning over a decades-long period.

In England, the government has a healthy lifestyle program it offers to people at high risk for cardiovascular disease with dismal results. It is the English Longitudinal Study of Ageing. One-third decline to enroll, 40% refused screening, 70% sporadically attend, and high dropout rates complete the picture. Goodness! Why is people's non-compliance a serious problem? Stop, Breathe, Think, Then act—long term. The goal of this book is to emphasize the benefits of constructive actions and attitudes—long term.

The American automobile industry a while back took a nosedive; this was the time when Japan excelled because adults in America thought short term and the Japanese considered the long term. Perhaps, that is why they are the longest-lived people on Earth. Aging is long-term by definition—period.

BARRIERS TO MOTIVATION

We used to believe that our genes determined our health. Many incorrectly continue to blame their genes. Big mistake. Now we know otherwise: how you live your life is the real foundation of your health (or lack thereof) and it plays a far greater role than your genetic history. A famous study of 2,872 Danish identical twin sets for almost three decades found that our genes' influence on health or disease is actually only 23% (females) to 26% (males).[1] That means that 74% to 77% (depending on your gender) of what affects your well-being is not genetic.

In other words, concerning your health, you're in the driver's seat. Your behavior determines most of your health and longevity—what I call your "health-span."

The worst, and fortunately not the most common, barriers are the "what the hell, that is my choice" choices. I have one intelligent friend who does not engage in physical activity, whose excuse is "I am too lazy." Another says, "I eat the way I do because I want to eat that way. Why not cash in a few years to eat what you want?"

Making choices you know are harmful is not wise. Choosing to disregard facts until it's too late is irresponsible. It is worse than playing roulette on a fixed table because you cannot win; instead, the bet is on how much you will lose! And it's not just years you lose; it's how you will exit life. Suffering from some undesirable illness which consumes your well-being and finances. Behaviors can have noteworthy influence on your health. Play at a health roulette table where the odds are only "how much benefit will this get me."

Assuming that it is too late for changes in your lifestyle to be effective is dead wrong. The HALE study (many of the larger, more important medical studies have names) found that death from heart attacks, the number one killer in America, could almost be eliminated (reduced by 73%) with a healthy lifestyle.[2] And this study *started with people 70 years and older*! For the remainder of the decade-long follow-up those who were active, had a good diet, did not smoke, and drank alcohol were one-sixth as likely to meet the number one killer face-to-face. I like the fact that alcohol was beneficial. Dean Martin, with his alcohol-based jokes, was my favorite comic.

In clinical medicine, a heart attack is a dreadful experience, among the worst pain and worry one can experience. Heart pain is not like other pain; it is pressure combined with the sensations of smothering and a feeling of looming death. It is commonly described as, "An elephant is standing on my chest." The punch line is you can choose to avoid it but you must start now.

Multiple other studies show that lifestyle benefits accrue no matter what period of your life you start. This dismisses the second great laggard myth: it is too late for a lifestyle change to benefit me. It is never too late; the Jerusalem Longitudinal Cohort Study showed significant benefits from start-ing an exercise program even as old as 85 years.[3] You don't have any valid reasons not to act. Get with the program.

As we will discuss in detail later, age-related diseases are common in people past middle age or even before. The disease must reach a certain threshold before making you sick. Therefore, and this is the take-home point, if you are well, stopping the disease you already have from progressing will keep you well. As we will discuss further, reversing, stopping, or even slowing the damage to your body before it is too advanced can delay or even avoid suffering.

JUST HOW IMPORTANT IS YOUR BODY?

Our bodies are our most important personal belongings. Yes, legally we own our bodies. We can give away a kidney today or at death donate a multitude of organs. Even convicts have the right to accept or refuse what is done to their bodies medically with the exception of forced feeding for hunger strikers. Recently, a death row inmate in Texas refused to take medication to restore sanity so his execution could legally proceed; it seems sanity is required (golly!); a judge ruled out forcible medication.

Our bodies are more valuable than money. Ask yourself what you would pay to be cured of a terminal illness such as cancer—your summer home, your BMW? The answer invariably is everything I have and all I can borrow, which perhaps is why pharmaceutical companies are developing drug treatments that cost over $1,000 a day! When faced with substantial health problems everything else rapidly becomes secondary. Our actions need to show that we realize health maintenance for suitable well-being is important before the tipping point is reached.

Yet, over 95% of all injuries and most illnesses are avoidable. Defensive driving courses are offered in most states and they must work. My insurance company reduces the collision premium when a customer becomes certified. Flu shots for the elderly will significantly decrease hospitalizations, flu-associated strokes, and deaths. According to the prestigious Centers for Disease Control, the average death from flu in America is 36,000, with 80% in the elderly (over 65). We all consider ourselves, sometimes to be invincible, doctors; yes doctors only get flu shots 40% of the time!! Get smart. Get with the program! You have everything to gain and nothing to lose.

The real dangers to humans are the diseases associated with aging: heart disease, stroke, cancer, Alzheimer's disease, and others. These too can be avoided with modest lifestyle modifications. But understanding how to take care of your body is important. Knowing what to put into it, knowing what to make it do, and what to avoid seems simple enough. Statistics scream but we seem to say so what, and we just go on. Not smart. Stop! Breathe! Think! Then Act!

HEALTH LITERACY IS THE HOLY GRAIL OF HEALTH

Almost every competent adult knows which behaviors are healthy and which are unhealthy, or do they? Two important studies show that half of American adults are health illiterate. In a national study of over 5,000 participants, only 16% were exercising regularly and consuming a healthy diet.[4] Declaring someone illiterate on any subject is an insult; it indicates desirable skills under a very low standard. The health illiterate have more emergency department visits and increased utilization of more expensive therapies. The study reaching those conclusions evaluated improper drug dosages, obtaining timely tests such as Pap smears, and understanding treatment instructions; as such, the studies evaluated health care literacy, not health literacy. I suspect true literacy concerning health fundamentals is much lower.

What is the relative value of different "literacies"? Important literacies include maintenance (reading, writing, and arithmetic), financial, cultural, social, and general knowledge. In the United States, the subsistence illiteracy rate is 1% and that is an important literacy to have but is reading as important as health—or finance? Stop! Breathe! Think! Then Act! About your health.

As confirmation of the value of health literacy, an English study of 7,857 subjects found that better health literacy was associated with 40% better survival.[5] When one's health or a loved one's health is seriously threatened, all other aspects of life become unimportant. Health will be discussed fully in chapter two, but the goal to maintain health and suffer fewer illnesses should drive our behaviors.

The health-promoting or disease-promoting behaviors are well known, so why are they ignored by a majority of the population? A dangerous, too often deadly paradigm obscures the lifestyle causation of chronic disease. Aging invariably causes serious diseases no matter what one's lifestyle, so enjoy life fully and get medical care to cure the disease when it comes.

A large part of a major disconnect between doing what is best for our health has to do with our brain's devaluation of future effects and overvaluation of the present. Dr. Eagleman, a neuroscientist at the Baylor College of Medicine where he directs the Laboratory for Perception and Action, has found the answers through scientific data. First, when offered chocolate cake, the more primitive parts of your brain crave the rich energy source of sugar, although other parts where rational thinking reside are concerned about the negative consequences.[6] In contrast, the paradigm for healthy lifestyle's benefits supposes that the benefits are decades away. He presents multiple studies that show people discount future benefits in favor of imme-diate rewards.

I don't exercise daily just to lengthen my life and prevent disability; those are important but distant benefits. There are perceptible proven benefits in the now. Mental functioning in older people measurably improved after work-out sessions[7] and so did life satisfaction in another study.[8] However, in both observations, the improvement was seen in those who were regulars, not from a single workout. Starting an exercise program requires commitment. In one study, only one of every six who started an exercise program remained com-mitted after a year.[9] If you are starting out, be gradual, not abrupt, in intensity and vow to continue for at least two months. Those who suspect health prob-lems should see their doctor beforehand.

There are factors promoting a sense of well-being brought on by any physi-cal activity, not just exercise: opioid production, self-image enhancement, and proof that personal physical performance remains intact are life-enhanc-ing benefits in the now. Although it may not be as apparent, the evidence is clear that regular exercise reduces blood pressure, improves the depressive symptoms of aging, and improves sleep. When I don't exercise for several days my sleep becomes less restful. Exercise is beneficial in people with sleep apnea beyond the weight loss earned.[10] We will examine this in more detail in a later chapter.

Thus, leading an active life enriches life as it is lived. It reduces the ravages of time and if implemented, even later in life, *can reverse what has been diminished that was valued.* Adopting healthy routines returns youthfulness; it turns back the clock. Having a positive body image need not be summar-ily dismissed as we age. A more positive attitude toward one's outlook is invaluable.

Wouldn't you like to be a member of the group who can look in the mirror and say, "not bad, I have aged well"? I went to a 50th high school reunion to receive a Hall of Fame Award (13th of 40,000 graduates) and, wow, were there ever differences in the way friends had aged! Those with more frequent exercise routines had a more positive body image as a reward. Internal aging is what benefits most from healthy lifestyles. I spoke to one alumnus who was a star athlete who became sedentary after college and had serious medical problems. Too bad.

Unfortunately, the aging of facial skin is primarily determined by exposure to sunlight rather than other behavioral factors. And some of us got a lot of sun in our youth.

Among aging-generated losses, decreased muscle mass and associated strength is important; mental competency is right up there and sexual dysfunction figures in as well, oh yes. Healthy lifestyles reduce losses in all three categories—significantly. Studies show that healthier men have less erectile dysfunction (ED). Moreover, studies took men with substantial ED who were inactive and started them on exercise programs; soon their sexual function improved.[11] Healthy behaviors yield rewards in the present, adding to life's enjoyment in the now. Serotonin is associated with mood, sleep, and mental functioning. It is increased by exercise, period.[12] Another mood-enhancing brain chemical is also increased with exercise.[13]

Apart from and just as important, psychological stress is part of aging. Depression of aging can tarnish the goldenness of the golden years. There is scientific evidence that not only are you composed of what you eat, what you eat influences how you think. In the Hordaland Health study, over 5,700 Norwegian adults were studied and those with more nutritious diets were less likely to be unhappy.[14] Also, higher intakes of processed foods increased anxiety! Tasting better does not translate to being better. We can train our taste. I cannot drink whole milk; it tastes greasy. Skim is my whim.

"Ageism" is the negative perception of aging, which encourages prejudicial attitudes toward older people; it can be present in all ages, especially in those who are suffering most from the ravages of aging. We have just mentioned the improvement of self-image from exercise but what about other people's image of you. Simulated descriptions of elderly men and women were reviewed by a large panel and those who were reported as more active were perceived more favorably than sedentary descriptions. Being more active triggers others to think more highly of you.

The American Cancer Society estimates, from the latest data, that over 42 million, or about one in seven adults, in the United States smoke cigarettes. This is down from almost half of adults smoking 40 years ago but considering the accumulation of warnings of tobacco's dangers and the escalating price, 42 million is shocking beyond belief.

When I was explaining the benefits of healthy living habits, a gentleman I met at a men's breakfast club meeting shocked me by announcing rather proudly that he was 80, had smoked cigarettes most of his life, and wasn't about to quit. I asked how he wished to die: continue to enjoy a functional life and exit rapidly or have a prolonged course of gradual deterioration? He changed his mind as I described the typical death from lung cancer. For a temporary enhancement of perception and mood from neurochemical release, a tobacco addict risks some of the most deadly, debilitating diseases known to medical science. Stop, Think, Act for the long term.

Barriers keeping older people from activity are feeble indeed. The number one is "too tired," closely followed by "lack of motivation" and "already active enough."[15] First, sedentary people are tired because of inactivity; "the use it or lose it" principle predominates biological systems. Keeping active preserves energy generation; becoming inactive is a negative feedback system, with which we must not allow ourselves to get involved. Reducing activity because we are tired results in more tiredness that reduces activity further. The lack of activity shrinks muscles (sarcopenia), weakening and furthering the detrimental process.

Over 5,000 participants in a national nutrition study were carefully examined for activity levels and healthy diets; only 16% (one out of six) had both. The key is the ability to delay gratification by impulse control. Having a calm rational approach to decision making promotes deferring rewards for a greater good, whereas emotional, impulsive bents are opposite in outcomes.

Deferred gratification experiments, done decades ago, have interesting results. Children who deferred gratification at an early age later had healthier lifestyles.[16] The ability to postpone temporary pleasures for a greater good later was a proxy for success in a variety of endeavors. Adults who exercise are more likely to defer immediate gratification for a longer-term goal.[17]

According to the National Institutes of Health (NIH), two-thirds of Americans are overweight (BMI > 24.9) and half of those overweight are obese (BMI > 30, 20% > ideal body weight) and these figures are increasing rapidly. The NIH website for accurately calculating BMI is http://www.nhlbisupport.com/bmi/.

Obesity is associated with more strongly valuing the now for rewards rather than future rewards.[18] My bride has a helpful attitude for avoiding overeating. "It gives me more pleasure to maintain looking good than the pleasure a high calorie diet would give."

Childhood obesity is a frightening statistic having tripled over 30 years to over one in five children. I did a study on younger patients (less than 50 years) having heart surgery for hardening of the arteries. Initially they did well because of less co-morbidity but their long-term outcomes were much worse than patients whose onset of disease occurred decades later. Obese children are at early risk for serious health problems. The health goal should be to delay the progression of chronic diseases and to "live long and prosper."

The metabolism of an obese person differs. Fat (adipose) cells differ from other cells. They have a little sliver of a nucleus because they only function as biological warehouses and a cellophane-like cell membrane that swells proportionately to body fat as they get fatter. We don't add more fat cells; the fat cells we have are grown bigger to hold the added fat. Although hard to accumulate in prehistoric times, body fat was highly desirable because our ancestors literally lived hand-to-mouth. The methods of husbandry were in infancy at risk to the harsh wiles of nature and preservation was unknown.

In addition, today, we don't understand the importance of salt in medieval life; it made spoiling food palatable. But before agriculture, body fat allowed endurance of periods of starvation, especially in childbearing females.

Evolution "selected" those who consumed parts of animals and plants containing higher calories, especially fat. So, genetically, we humans like to consume fatty high-energy foods and lots of salt. Our distant ancestors had to walk great distances as hunter-gatherers to obtain food and they sweat which loses salt. Whereas now, for our food we stand in line at the grocery and obtain foodstuffs from around the world. Our attitudes must change or our health will suffer.

Behaviors that allowed us to survive persist as irrational choices in a different world—the world of now. In the world of plenty, the behavior of stuffing ourselves is no longer a primitive survival plan; it sets the stage for some of the worst diseases.

An obese person risks some of the most deadly, debilitating diseases known to medical science. Diabetes and its many complications, arthritis, heart and vascular disease, and various cancers are mainly located in the pelvic area—rectal, prostate, cervical, uterine, and others. Stop, Breathe, Think, then Act for the long term.

Indisputable scientific evidence continues to mount which concludes that a diet rich with fruits and vegetables reduces the plagues of aging—heart disease and cancer. There is benefit toward reduction of Alzheimer's disease and Parkinsonism as well. Such a diet with the addition of liberal amounts of olive oil and moderate amounts of red wine is designated the "Mediterranean diet" which is considered one of the utmost health-promoting diets. Three-fourths of Americans prefer to avoid eating a healthy diet. Instead they consume high-caloric animal fats and have achieved the highest rate of obesity in the world.

If we were satisfied with three or even four decades of quality life, lifestyle transgressions would be inconsequential but we want more. No one wants to spend the last decades of life lacking vitality, or in pain, or both continuing to an early death. In almost four decades of medical practice, I have never seen a patient who detects the reaper's chariot landing next to their bed who does not pray to God and ask their physician to pull them back from the abyss. Everyone wants to stick around at least to observe their grandchildren become adults and perhaps even to hold a great-grandchild and realize your genes will truly outlive you.

These obviously destructive lifestyles hurry our physical deterioration; why do we embrace them? Because we don't Stop, Breathe, Think, and then Act. All the danger is vaguely distant but it is real! Make a list of your greatest personal fears: Losing your job, becoming destitute, being displaced from your home, enduring incontestable public humiliation, or becoming imprisoned are some major dreadful events. But none rivals being told you must endure terminal disease's illnesses that cannot be effectively treated. Once that happens, everything else suddenly doesn't matter.

You can even affect the aging of your cells! Cellular age can be determined by looking at the ends of chromosomes (telo-meres, end-stuff in Greek). A study that measured telomere health of several thousand identical twin sets found that when one twin had exercised more during the previous 12 months, his cells were significantly younger than those of his twin.[19] This phenomenal benefit from exercise is even more pronounced in older individuals.[20]

Those of us lucky enough to grow old will most likely encounter illness; as the body ages, certain anatomical functions will decline; it is inevitable. The message of this book is that we can avoid debilitating disease; we can live longer; and those extra decades can be good ones full of life. But to achieve it, we need to Stop, Breathe, Think, then Act.

What I learned about health and disease in my 35 years as a cardiovascular surgeon convinces me that we need to embrace a "free will" concept of health. Each of us will get what they resolve to get through chosen behaviors. That perspective is the only way to live long, and prosper (i.e., be successful in aging). Aging without getting old is the goal. Specifically, I mean that predetermination, which we prohibit in every other aspect of our lives, needs to be operative in the manifestation of our health.

Chapter 2

Celebrating the Leaven of Life—Health

How to Find It and Keep It

UNDERSTANDING HEALTH BETTER

Why do we not understand the essentials of health better? We neglect health because we too often loosely grasp the most important things in our life as knee-jerk responses, without thinking; they just happen. Health is the water in our swimming pool, being the one most important thing, without which it would not be a swimming pool. Our lives are filled by important events and we concentrate on them, not on what allows them to take place. But what allows these important events to take place simply happens. We don't have to think about going up the stairs; we concentrate on what we will do when we get to the top. We pay attention to the solid material of our "pool" (our body), not the life it contains—overlooking the essential thing. We ignore its importance because, as the water in our swimming pool, it is just there. We use our health to do things. We think about the things that our body allows us to do. Think about the essential part—your living body.

Accordingly, health is the most cherished and least understood human condition; it is appreciated mostly when impaired, which is a very twisted notion; that faulty concept is definitely hazardous to well-being. An old song catches the mood and illustrates the faulty thinking, entitled "You never miss the water, till the well runs dry." There has been a lot of talk lately about the perilous world situation and the upshot is that one cannot deal satisfactorily with something that they do not understand. People claim to understand important lifestyle subjects such as health until asked to define them; then they invariably cast health as the opposite of disease. Health is that but much, much more.

Every adult will experience serious threats to their health and those frightful experiences rapidly eclipse all other worldly concerns. Compared to serious illness, all other difficulties are secondary. We must recognize the great value of health. If you ask people a hypothetical question to determine their value of health, the answer is consistent and should not surprise. "If you were diagnosed with a terminal illness and a possible cure was available, how much would you pay? Would you give up one of your two cars?" The answer always is I would pay all I have and all I could borrow. Serious threats to our health are more crucial than our material possessions, by far.

The word "health" derives from Old English roots meaning wholeness or the state of being uninjured. Originally, the word meant "being fit" for life—having health was a good omen for all of one's activities; close to hale, which has persisted unchanged as meaning to be strong. Health, however, currently has abridged to mean freedom from physical maladies. As defined in this chapter, the good news is that there is much more to health.

The World Health Organization defines health as: "A state of complete physical, mental and social well-being and not merely the absence of disease or infirmity." Health worsens with illness, yet is incompletely defined by absence of disease that defines minimalist or subsistence health. Instead, the army's slogan "the best you can be" applies to each individual's state of health and "best in spirit" should define the concept of health. Social, mental, physical, and even spiritual states of health or wellness of functioning can be improved and a healthy self-assurance promotes behaviors to improve functioning. The more you use it, the more you boost it.

Throughout recorded history, starting from Hippocrates two and a half millennia ago, medicine has focused on restoring health by treating illness-caused-by-disease and patients are prompted to seek medical attention when they sense that their well-being has changed. But counter to a very pervasive paradigm, subsistence health is not "all there is."

Attaining health well beyond absence of disease should be our focus. Health is much more than absence of pain. A quadriplegic has interrupted neurological pathways, which prevent painful sensations below the neck, and no one would consider the condition healthy. Pain is not an enemy; it is an important protective mechanism that keeps from getting ulcers of the skin. Diabetics who have lost sensation in the feet are prone to get damage because their body does not tell them to change positions.

WHAT EXACTLY IS HEALTH?

Above all else, health is a gauge of functionality; it is loosely termed "fitness." Health increases or decreases as a person's ability to function changes. That is the healthy concept of health. Athletes and soldiers undergo rigorous physical training to improve physical fitness. I was never as physically healthy as I was when in the military.

Students and professionals spend considerable time developing and honing mental skills. I was never as mentally healthy as I was when in medical school. Ordinary health-conscious people exercise in gyms and neighborhoods to improve or maintain physical health and by reading and doing puzzles for mental health.

Many of our daily activities are not done for pay; they are fun but more important such activities maintain and even augment our health. Remaining active in ways that challenge is the key. Years ago, before modern managed care, patients remained at bed rest after surgical procedures for prolonged periods because it was considered necessary for healing. Some died unnecessarily from blood clots to the lungs and pneumonia. Still prolonged bed rest is deadly. Occasionally, on long airline flights, people can develop blood clots in their legs. It is wise to get up and walk the aisle every hour or so when permissible.

As humans evolved, the ability to travel further in foraging for food, which was definitely a survival benefit for hunter-gatherers. Survival benefits evolve genetically and increased activity's possible harm is eliminated by chemical changes which explains benefit from physical exertion. The ancients were opportunistic feeders because food was often scarce bestowing advantages to the more mobile. In addition, mankind killed prey and enemies initially by throwing objects, so evolution would have favored those having greater fitness with hand-eye coordination who hunted in packs. To cooperate in hunting in packs required socialization, so health involved socialization as well.

Health is qualitative and divisible into different aspects. Because the majority of threats to health are physical or mental in nature, those aspects are considered the primary determinants of health. Rosy cheeks, muscular build, pleasant countenance, and energetic behaviors are superficial evidence of physical health. Mental, emotional, social, occupational, and spiritual health aspects are important as well.

TYPES OF HEALTH

Physical health is the easiest to reconcile. If I can perform better bodily actions, to that extent, I am physically healthier. Each year, we can watch athletes trying out for the National Football League (NFL) run, jump, and demonstrate agility on TV. Those who are physically healthier are more likely to be recruited. We demonstrate our physical health each day by what actions we can do or not do. Our physical abilities largely determine the lifestyle we must lead, especially as we age. Life can be a sprint across a field or a cage we can choose in which to reside. Doing brings about doing more, physically and mentally and emotionally and socially.

To understand emotional health we must understand emotions. We receive a lot of information and must classify it according to importance. All humans laugh, get angry, cry, and love without being taught to do so. Emotions are genetic impositions. Emotions are part of the brain classified as mammalian. It is part and parcel of why the mammal class dominates the Earth. Emotions are a survival attribute. Imagine a prehistoric humanoid hearing a saber-tooth tiger growl. The response would differ whether the tiger was outside your cave, outside the tribe's perimeter, or across the river at a hostile tribe's camp. Our emotions filter information through personalization. The more personal, the more valuable is the subject. What is more personal than your BODY?

Mental health becomes important when severely impaired, especially in regard to very recent memory. We need to know what we did within the last half hour. Did we take our meds? Did we turn off the stove? Our independent living depends on recent memory. Our hippocampus (hippo) is a small part of our brain that keeps us independent. It weighs about the same as a nickel (5 grams) and besides recent memory it tells us where we are so we don't get lost. It shrinks in late adulthood, which is why we may go into a room and forget what we were seeking. Its decreased functioning explains why people with dementia get lost. It is important to protect our hippos and we can do so. Erickson used CAT scans to measure the hippos of older people and found exercise not only stopped the shrinkage, it increased hippo's size when exercise was started.[1] More is better.

Recognition that improving performance enhances health empowers individuals to improve their health status. Although superficially one may consider health only physical, there are several categories of health in addition to physical health including intellectual, educational, perceptual, emotional, spiritual, and financial. All of the different aspects interact. Deteriorating physical health affects emotional health adversely and the opposite occurs. Educational health promotes intellectual health and educational status impacts physical health as well as financial status.

The vast majority of our behavior is habit. It makes good sense to establish habits that contribute to our functionality, especially as we age. My bride was an apprentice chef at Commander's Palace and then went to law school. Over the years, she developed ways of keeping flavor in dishes while reducing fat and calories. Now, when we go out to eat, we must be careful not to eat too much fat or our bodies actually suffer. We feel bloated and uncomfortable.

A fatty meal makes one mentally sluggish. Remember watching your relatives fall asleep watching football after a big thanksgiving meal? We might have changed our eating habits, but do we feel that we have given up pleasure? No, we enjoy eating just as much as before and we allow ourselves rare, moderate indulgences. These excesses are much more appreciated than when they were routine and are not missed.

"Health" is the overused word for well-being. It includes safety, comfort, and good fortune. As mentioned, it has a variety of facets: physical health is the most talked about, followed closely by mental health; however, we all appreciate that health can have social, financial, educational, and emotional aspects too. These are the determinants of what our mind tells us our state of well-being is.

None of the aspects of health stand alone; they interact—enhancing or diminishing one another. For the most part, aspects of well-being improve or diminish in parallel, meaning the best approach to maximize health is all-embracing. Benjamin Franklin was a very accomplished writer, scientist, and diplomat who was a co-founder of the United States. In his remarkable autobiography, Franklin outlines how he came to greatness, which he calls: "The Bold and Arduous Project of Arriving at Moral Perfection." He concentrated distinctly on improving 13 qualities and graded his adherence until he established a habit. He then moved on to forming the next good habit. Franklin's method is good for promoting health. Since 99% of behavior is habit, we should set a goal of forming beneficial habits.

An athlete is physically healthier than a sedentary individual. An acclaimed professor is educationally healthier than an uneducated person. However, illustrating the different parameters, the uneducated individual may or may not be healthier emotionally. It is important to understand the different aspects of health to attain it fully.

Physical and mental levels of functioning increase from childhood and peak at different periods of adult life and then have a slow decline. Physical strength and endurance peak in late teens and early twenties but decline can be delayed by continued efforts. The average NFL tenure is six seasons. Brett Favre retired for the last time as a professional quarterback at 41 years of age. Bret was in remarkable shape as he aged. Scientific data inevitably shows that increasing physical activity results in increasing physical functionality benefiting physical health.

HOW MUCH IS TOO MUCH?

Most everything is best in moderation; increases all should be gradual in exercise to avoid injuries. Very few achieve the level of physical health to play professional sports; those are the neuro-muscular geniuses. And often overall physical health of those chosen few stays marvelous for a short period. I became friends with an all-pro professional football player because our children attended the same school. He had starred for the Jets before injuries ended his career. During meetings, he could sit only for short periods because of back spasms and would have to stand but because of knee injuries, he would have to sit after a few minutes. I followed him about the room, grateful that I had never had the talent to be so injured.

A major misconception originated from the consideration of the brain and body as a machine, which as a purely engineering comparison is correct, but although our body obeys mechanical laws, it is structurally biological and functions mechanically. Machines wear out giving them a mantra: "Use it and lose it." Differently than purely mechanical systems, biological systems constantly repair their wear, cell by cell; cells that die are constantly replaced according to the extent the body determines according to usage. The mantra changes to "Use it or lose it." Actually, the more you use your body, the more you boost it. WOW.

We all know from experience that as we do something physically or mentally, we become better at it. "But this was when I was young," you protest. No, laws of nature remain the same. Although the older body may take longer to mend. You will regain whatever you lose by doing; otherwise, there would be no reason for physical therapy and rehab.

This brings us to another health axiom: the secret of health is how much is enough, and the secret of disease is how much is too much. A Chinese proverb exemplifies this point: "A knife honed to its sharpest will dull soon." Lifetime health especially the physical aspect is not a sprint; it is an ultramarathon. Slow balanced improvement would be best but one must be careful not to overdo. This is recommended for those of us who are average; there is no scientific evidence that elite endurance athletes suffer from their extremes.

WHAT SHOULD YOUR HEALTH GOALS BE?

The important lesson of aging is to maintain a quality of life, which should be one's goal. Realizing one's quality of life means being able to do the things one wants to do self-sufficiently. Running in the park, traveling and vacationing, gardening, managing your affairs, interacting with others meaningfully, attending reunions or religious services, going out for a night or to a sporting event—these are the kinds of activities that add quality to life.

How Does Your Brain Stay Healthy?

Functioning is our essential necessity. Mental functioning peaks later and lasts longer than physical health but obeys the same principles. Medicine previously considered that humans were born with all the brain cells (neurons) they would ever have and that neurons were inevitably and continually dying in an aging brain. This has proven erroneous: brains make new cells, although the slow production does not replace at the rate neurons die, especially in certain areas of the brain. There are behaviors we will explore that promote growth and decrease attrition of neurons.

A healthy functioning mind does not only depend on the number of neurons in a particular brain. Although, the average three-pound brain has 100 billion neurons. It is mostly how the present neurons function. Neurons are unique in that they are gregarious cells. Put a single neuron in a Petri dish outside the body and it will soon deteriorate and die. Instead, place a group of separated individual neurons in a Petri dish and they will seek each other out, join, and thrive. Neurons communicate with each other by touching their appendages called dendrites. They have processes, which reach out and connect similar to shaking hands. Mental exercise creates more neuron handshaking. Neuron handshaking is what provides mental functioning.

The neuronal network is analogous to Facebook—there are huge numbers of participants that can connect or not connect—it depends on their inclinations. Learning causes or is the result of forming new additional connections and disuse presumably results in disconnections. The dynamics allow rehabilitation of brain injury from strokes or trauma; new connections form to replace those destroyed.

As mentioned, decreasing mental activity over time results in the atrophy of mental functioning and increasing mental activity improves mental health. Just as repetitive physical exercises successively allows lifting of greater weights and becoming stronger, repetitive mental processes increase speed and accuracy. Mental health functioning benefits perhaps even more from new activities as well as repeating the same mental tasks.

Emotional health is important as people age. Chronic depression is an unwholesome emotional state that can be delayed or lessened by social and physical activity. It has been said that the first half of our lives is spent gathering and the last half in giving up what we gathered. As we age, many areas of functioning we prized gradually are given back. Non-acceptance of this reality can be a problem. I can no longer work all night and be fresh in the morning. The amount of turmoil one experiences in acceptance of lifestyle changes depends on the individual. The important aspect is that I no longer need to work all night on carrying for sick or injured people. I am able to do what I need to do and that is good. Each of us should judge our health status on the basis of whether or not we are able to function well enough to live a good life.

A beloved aunt who looked much younger than her age was very active in every area of life, but had periods of deep depression from overconcern from every symptom she experienced. She would take to bed for long periods and constantly call me for reassurance. She lived to be 97 and died during her sleep—illness-free. A substantial part of her life was lessened with disease worry. When I asked why she doted on negatives, it seemed to be because she had been so vibrant, sought-after, and continued to value those aspects without readjustment to reality.

My mother had many serious illnesses and reacted realistically or even stoically. She once had a serious stroke and lay in her kitchen until a neighbor found her after several days. When I visited her in the hospital, she gave me a crooked smile, extended her good hand, and said with slurred speech, "You don't know how hard your kitchen floor is until you lay on it for a few days." She tackled rehab with a vengeance demanding double the normal hours in therapy and would get orderlies and me to assist her in walking the halls with the support of a wheelchair between therapies.

She got a friend to transport her home against medical advice and recovered with scarcely a limp. She managed a 130-acre ranch and rental properties, traveled, and drove herself around until the last few years of her life. Illness and aging have considerable variability but can always be magnified or lessened by the bearer's mind-set.

As we go into the phase of becoming into our so-called golden years, we must readapt just as we did in adolescence—to a different role. Then we transitioned from childhood to adulthood and noted the different ways people viewed us. Now we transition from middle age to seniorhood and must accept the reality that we are viewed differently. We can adopt ageism's disapproval and think negatively, which is untrue, or as history dictates: We the elderly are valuable because of our experiences and our contributions and a continuing purpose.

To paraphrase the Biblical parable: "to those given much less will seem to be taken away. To those given little even that they have will be taken." The parable goes on—germane to our discussion—the amount taken depends on what was done with what was originally given. Use it or lose it is biologically true.

Our bodies have marvelous repair mechanisms but are similar to our first responder organizations; they must have regular drills and maintenance. Being active mentally and physically assures that your body can respond and repair itself, and this maintenance keeps your functioning intact.

AVOIDING DISTRACTIONS

Depression is a shroud that makes everything seem worse than it is. The wearer gladly wears it. Happiness is the flip side of depression which cannot coexist. Thus, depression must be mollified and measures to do so are available. Happiness' main theory is the "set point theory" which is dependent in large measure on expectations. Everyone determines personal standards which when met or exceeded are satisfying and, contrarily, when unmet are depressing. Set point theory explains why wealth does not assure happiness and ward off depression. As one accumulates more, expectations require even more for satisfaction.

A game show named "Deal or No Deal" illustrates the phenomena well. Contestants start with 20-odd briefcases that contain prizes ranging from 1¢ to a million dollars. As the game progresses, depending on their choices, the amount of winnings changes, as does their mood. As they get more, they want more, even to risk everything they have won. The show is the only example where a contestant can be unhappy after winning hundreds of thousands of dollars because the million escaped.

Emotional health is a balance between perceptions of what is and expectations. Expectations must change to match reality as a person ages. This requires acceptance of things that cannot be changed and fortitude ("stick with it" mind-set, one of the original virtues of Plato) to change the important things for the better.

Spiritual health and emotional health characterize a Venn diagram of overlap between two areas. Spiritual is not taken to suggest religiosity or the existence or absence of a soul. Spiritual health is an inner peace from concern for higher matters. It is a realization of finitude and that as a part of the physical universe there is something in what we inhabit that far exceeds us and, most importantly, come to terms with that something. It is a non-physical part of personhood which is core to the personality—values, beliefs, morals, and conscience—which only surfaces into consciousness when asked about; otherwise unconsciously what I prefer to call spirit nudges the consciousness to act in a certain way. And unconsciously, spirit punishes well-being when its nudgings are not followed.

Spirit is not emotional but uses emotions to reward or punish. Theology offers solutions and promises which may instruct or even fulfill one's spiritual health paradigm. Naturalistic atheism may satisfy others. Whatever one's choice of path, a profundity accompanies acceptance of what is and what is to be. All things with a beginning must have an ending; such is the way of life. Lack of spiritual health carries many fears which erode well-being.

Social health must be cultivated and is not something, as it often appears to be, discretionary in life. Occupation and energy of youth is more conducive to social connections. Social health overlaps with physical, mental, and especially emotional health, serving to improve each area. Just like neuronal connections, social connections are plentiful if pursued. Most religious institutions, clubs, charitable organizations, and alma maters offer social opportunities.

Visiting neighbors and even talking to strangers are chances to connect and improve social health. Isolation is not a sought-after human good. Humans are genetically programmed as social animals. Imagine hominids even before cave dwelling; there were no guns, no real fangs or claws, and human athleticism was and still is no match for predators. Our salvation and dominance came from tribal pack-hunting where the many would attack an animal several times our size from different angles throwing rocks and other objects, making us evolve into the best killers the world has ever known. Socialization remains important today lest we wither like the lone nerve cell.

A scientific study is not needed to determine which direction a rock will fall when tossed out a window. And although there are ample studies in the past that show tremendous benefits of exercise, it is common sense that if more is done, more benefits will be realized. Athletes do not merely show up for game day. They repetitively simulate maneuvers they will perform during competition so their strength, speed, and agility are developed to their peak. For superior intellectual health, professors toil for years, sometimes an entire career, incrementally refining a concept. Einstein spent years on his theories going over and over the same thoughts. Great athletes and intellectuals finally attain peak health but in a single aspect. Health obeys the laws of specificity. For optimum health, one needs to attend to all aspects of health.

Everyone should have the same health goals on a lesser scale: perform activities that fine-tune functionality and, thus, augment their health. As mentioned, for physical activities, strength, speed, and agility count. For mental activities, mastery of complexity, accuracy, and efficiency count.

The undeniable message is that health can be improved by efforts that improve functionality and the witticism "use it or lose it" applies. Everything requires effort; nothing magically appears. Leibniz's explanation is "the principle of sufficient reason." Health obeys the principle of sufficient reason. A man able to accomplish astounding physical feats, Jack LaLanne, fitness guru, was able to do so because of fitness efforts. Jack at 70 years of age swam and towed 70 rowboats, with passengers, against strong currents, handcuffed and shackled, for a mile in San Diego Harbor. Health and its desirable functionally are directly proportional to our efforts to increase function.

Consider the question: If you could live to 150 years of age and have one aspect of your health remain young, which aspect would you choose? Would you want to inhabit a body with an alert mind aware of a feeble likely painful body? Or would it be desirable to occupy a vigorous physique but a mind unable to make use of it? Few on reflection would choose to live two lifetimes under those conditions. Contrarily, what if one could maintain both an alert mind and a vigorous physique? One can. Read on.

Medical science can educate as to how to avoid disease and what constitutes a "healthy lifestyle" but even in that important role, medicine is mainly concerned with treating disease. Western medicine, especially in the United States, pays lip service to preventative medicine. Preventative medicine training programs for doctors exist but are focused on public health issues, not an individual's health.

Preventative measures in public health deal with maintaining health of populations by preventing disease. Some measures considered are vaccinations, condom use, and hand washing. Worldwide prevention focuses on clean water, malnutrition, poverty, and basic needs. These measures are vitally important but are not the main health issues facing adults in America. In the developed world and the rest, most health concerns are lifestyles determined by individuals.

Understanding health benefits from behavior is a diamond of great value with multiple important facets and the various degrees of healthiness within each depends on functionality. Health is not fixed at one level; it can be improved or diminished by behaviors. It can be dangerously diminished through illnesses from diseases. Most chronic diseases are long-standing, taking a long time to effect our health and can be slowed or reversed by stopping unhealthy behaviors or substituting healthy behaviors. Since disability and death from chronic diseases steadily increase as we age, healthy aging should be our goal. Successful aging replaces disability with functionality.

Healthy aging is aging that preserves functional capacity. We are saturated with newly minted health books on proper ways to exercise, eat, interact, and manage our lives better; and some even work, for a while. Most are instruments that make one feel better because something is being done. Feeling better is satisfying but to be of consequence, the changes must continue for decades. In decades, healthy lifestyles have remarkable results.

Our bodies are the ultimate and only places we have to live. Realizing that one can be master or slave of their body is the initial step of healthy aging. Incremental improvements in each of the areas of health are keys to success. Attaining and retaining health is a long-term process. Public gymnasiums fill considerably after each New Year's resolution period, reverting to the regulars by March.

Proof of healthy functionality extended far beyond what is expected in America by adopting vital lifestyles resides in the enclaves of exceptionally healthy, long-lived people—termed "Blue Zones." The National Geographic Society commissioned Dan Buettner to study people in these sites around the world and determine their secrets of long, healthy living. In contrast to what would be considered true by Americans, there is mostly a negative correlation with wealth. In four of the five Blue Zones, residents there are poorer than their surrounding less-healthy neighbors. Paradoxically, moderate poverty in the Blue Zones forces people into healthier lifestyles. This of course is augmented by cultural emphasis of healthy behaviors. These include: active physical work (necessity), diets high in plant foods and low in animal protein (costs less), reduced caloric intake (plant foods), religiosity, and socialization (limited technology).

Blue Zone's residents emphasize lifestyle effects on healthy aging. The rates of Blue Zone centenarians are 30 or more times the average among Americans. Dan Buettner met an 80-year-old man in a Blue Zone in Costa Rica for an interview at 7:00 a.m., who wanted to go to his mother's house. They borrowed bicycles, peddling down a dirt road where his mother, over a hundred years of age, gladly met them. She had been up since 4:00 a.m. and had prayed, gathered eggs from the chicken coop, drew water from the well for coffee, ground corn by hand, and had a breakfast of eggs, coffee, and tortillas. Using a machete, she had cleared the bush around her house. The son, an 80-year-old great-grandfather, sat like a son and listened to his mother. Wouldn't you like to experience that kind of later life? MARVELOUS.

Don't be fooled by thinking that in these small isolated Blue Zone areas genetic uniformity is causal. There is a Blue Zone in the Los Angeles area, Loma Linda home of the Adventists. Their religious convictions, not poverty, motivate their dedication to live healthier. Dan Buettner describes charming encounters with self-sufficient centenarians still enjoying life. They were socializing with their families and friends, gardening, chopping firewood, and looking forward fully to living each day. They were religious people retaining their purpose for living each day, free from the major disabilities and infirmities that the rest of the world accepts as inevitable because their lifestyles make it happen.

The goal of this chapter and this book is to convince readers they are responsible for their health. They can make an important difference in their well-being with realistic efforts. Since what one does not know does not exist to them and what one does not know about health can kill; health literacy is the first step in achieving a healthier status.

Chapter 3

Keeping Alive

Vital Keys of Age-Related Disease

WHAT DOES AGING HAVE TO DO WITH DISEASE?

"Aging" is definitely not a four-letter word, unless you make it so. Don't go there. Aging lets us go from childhood as incompetent parasitic charmers to beings in control of our worlds. We come into life as the weakest, most vulnerable creatures on Earth. As we aged from infancy, we built pyramids and went to the moon. Aging of premium wine makes it better and it is so with humans. The destroyer of aging's gifts is the disease that can become attached.

Disease is the enemy of well-being and can limit functional independence. Dis-ease, meaning a lack of ease, is a condition having a host of implications—all bad—because disease reduces the level of well-being. According to *Stedman's Medical Dictionary*, a disease produces "an interruption, cessation, or disorder of bodily function." But the interval a disease takes from its beginning to when decreases in function occur is very important, as we shall see.

In medical schools, you might think that the major emphasis is on studying disease and its prevention—not so. The emphasis is on how to diagnose and treat disease, which seems the correct approach because medicine's job is to diagnose and treat disease. Those who want to concentrate on the study of disease become pathologists.

In doing heart artery surgery, I recognized the importance of diet in preserving the new arteries I created. The staff made an appointment with a dietician for whoever prepared the meals for the patients after heart surgery. I recognized that an expert was needed as I explained the importance to patients and their families. "The consultation and your compliance will make my work look good," I explained, usually to their amusement.

When defining the status of one's health as the ability to function, disease sketchily emerges as a distinct diminishment of functioning. A decline of functioning heralds an illness. Think of the last time a "cold" made you a bed-ridden cougher. That was not bad as age-related diseases because your body and some meds had you back in health in a few days. Age-related disease is usually an entirely different scenario, the illness doesn't just go away and the damage to functionality may be permanent. It is important to note that much of the chronic diseases' treatments are designed to reduce the illnesses. The diseases often remain elusive. Cancer is the sole exception as it is treated directly but all too many cancers recur.

Producing pain is a common way the body diminishes one's ability to function. Pain signals that one should rest to allow healing. Another way the body signals to take it easy is generally feeling bad (malaise) usually having a distinct lack of energy. Most pain, especially chronic pain, is caused by inflammation which is why a class of meds reducing pain work by interrupt-ing inflammation. Aspirin and other over-the-counter meds are of that class. Narcotics do not go to the root cause; they attach to receptors in the brain and spinal cord reducing the nerve transmission announcing pain. This effect tends to give pleasure, especially if taken when pain is not being experienced, so narcotics are addictive.

There are three recognized criteria to define a disease: (1) a specific causal agent (usually a bacteria or virus); (2) identifiable symptoms and signs; (3) specific anatomical alterations. Any two of these criteria define a disease.

Specific anatomic alterations can be visible to the unaided eye such as a rash or when using a microscope to examine various tumorous tissues. Under the microscope, tumor cells are not uniform in size and lack the organization of normal tissue allowing a specific diagnosis—such as lung cancer or colon cancer. The microscopic diagnoses are almost always specific. On the other hand, non-specific changes such as skin rashes may have multiple causes and are not as helpful in diagnosing diseases.

HOW DO THE WORDS "ILLNESS" AND "DISEASE" DIFFER?

Although the two words appear interchangeable, "illness" differs from "disease." Their difference is very important in chronic disease. Illness signals worsened health recognized by decreased functionality. Illnesses prompt patients to seek relief through medical technology. Since multiple diseases may cause a single illness, diagnosticians identify the causal disease to treat its illness correctly. Diagnoses of diseases are labels to allow correct treatment. Illnesses, not diseases, and not physicians, are medicine's cost-drivers.

Diseases are broadly divided into those rapidly producing illness's symptoms as rapid (acute) or slow (chronic). This is a foundational concept of this book. Almost every disease has a latent period during which the body mounts a reaction to a harmful agent. Poisonings are a good example of the exceptions.

When you go out in public and someone sneezes contaminating the air with flu viruses, the virus enters your body but it usually takes several days or weeks—the latent period—before the virus multiplies and your body responds, making you ill.

Acute diseases relatively rapidly cause illnesses (within six weeks), allowing them to be accurately diagnosed and usually effectively cured. Differing considerably, chronic diseases often take decades to produce illnesses, which usually require recurring treatments. Frequently, chronic diseases masquerade as benign conditions with sudden, often catastrophic illnesses. Examples are strokes and heart attacks. Patients are well one minute and gravely ill the next. The aim of most treatment regimens of chronic diseases is to reduce the illnesses.

Causal agents of common acute diseases are most often infectious such as bacteria and viruses. Robert Hooke, an English genius, made one of the most important inventions in determining medical disease causation: the microscope. The microscope is invaluable in diagnosing disease as well but it diagnoses more than it determines causality.

In acute disease the cause is apparent, whereas in chronic disease the cause is not always clear. As an example, high cholesterol does not cause heart disease; it is an "associated factor" termed medically as a "risk factor." Lowering cholesterol produces less vascular disease; it does not eliminate the problem. The medical literature is chockfull of studies showing that elevated cholesterol is a risk factor. One of the early studies could not be repeated today. Two Finnish mental institutions were assigned a regular diet or a low cholesterol diet for six years and the deaths from heart disease were significantly higher in the regular diet institution. They then switched diets and observed for another six years and the figures reversed.

Relation of age to chronic disease is because the longer one lives, the greater chance that they will have these diseases. In other words, living produces diseases from accumulation of the damage of living. Chronic diseases are age-related and, more importantly, lifestyle-related.

DISEASES ACCORDING TO CAUSES

Distinguishable symptoms (what patients experience) and signs (what doctors detect) define illnesses that result from disease and if the aggregate is unique enough, it satisfies one of the criteria defining a disease. Obvious patterns are termed "syndromes." Syndromes often are named for their discoverers, the anatomical area affected, or the general pathological process. Some have acronyms such as acquired immunodeficiency syndrome (AIDS). There are thousands of syndromes, many of which are unknown outside a particular medical specialty or because they are so rare. As a professional healer, you have arrived when you have a syndrome named after you.

It is important to emphasize that most illnesses can result from a number of different diseases. The disease causing an illness can simply be recognizable as a simple disease such as influenza or a more complex syndrome. The majority of diseases are not recognized as syndromes; they are diagnosed from knowing the cluster of diseases that cause specific symptoms. Then the medical diagnostician considers the list of diseases for an illness, picks the most likely ones, and orders tests if needed to identify specifically the cause of the illness.

Causal agents may be simple straightforward agents or they may be complex. Influenza viruses that cause flu are examples of obvious causal agents. These tiny living things are so incomplete biologically; they enter living cells like terrorists, take over the cellular DNA, and order it to construct more viruses. Then they destroy the host cell as they exit.

The cause of arteriosclerosis (literally, artery hardening) is obscure because it is secondary to a number of factors that damage the lining of arteries with superimposition of a harmful healing process. Arteriosclerosis is more common in people with hypertension, elevated cholesterol, family history of early vascular disease, obesity, and in males but these are not the causes, so they are termed "associated factors."

Even in the case of a disease that has a known cause, the cause does not have to be identified. Dr. Michael Gottleib of University of California at Los Angeles (UCLA) noticed that gay patients were appearing with rare diseases caused by deficient immune systems in 1981 and it became a well-described and feared disease before isolation of the HIV virus two years later—AIDS.

Anatomical alterations are recognizable changes in normal bodily structure. These changes may be seen without a microscope as in a reddened strep throat on physical examination but usually are positively identified from specially stained slides under a microscope. No single technological advance in medical history has added so much to understanding disease as the microscope.

Injuries are not diseases, although they can cause diseases. A wound can become infected. Bones can fail to heal. Various organs can fail when injured. Injuries produce acute illnesses. Injuries like chronic diseases become more common as one ages because deficiencies in balance predispose to falls and bodies weaken increasing susceptibility.

Thus, a physical or mental decline in well-being heralds illness. Illness manifests through symptoms that are "changes in normal structure, function, or sensation experienced by the patient." Patients who experience distressing symptoms go to physicians or other healthcare providers who diagnose the causal disease. As mentioned, a disease is not an illness; it is a label used to decide what to do about the illness.

Diseases and death rates have changed considerably over the past several millennia. The most reliable ancient longevity statistics are from Egyptian and Roman records. Over one of every four infants died. Sources report that men lived to be 25 to 30 years on average, while women and slaves died sooner. Alexander the Great certainly would have had access to the best available food and medical care but died at 32, from an infection. Infections were the most common cause of death, whereas now infections cause about 3% of American deaths. A century ago, American men, among the longest-lived on the planet, averaged dying at 52 years of age. This amounts to an increase of over 50%! And going forward it will better, especially with the proper management.

Plagues were often out of control until the last century. The "Black Death" plague in two years (1348–1350) killed over 100 million Europeans—about a third of the population. High mortality from infections and trauma kept most from reaching beyond late middle age when chronic diseases become important. Until the end of the nineteenth century compound fractures (when the bone ends pierce the skin) were treated by amputation, a solution that would be unconscionable today. Malaria several decades ago was the leading cause of death in the world. At the moment, malaria is not in the top ten. However, in poor countries, infections continue to cause one-third of fatalities but less than 5% in developed countries. Presently, because ancient scourges were eliminated, people live long enough for chronic diseases to be the main causes of death.

DISEASE MOSTLY IS FROM OUR OWN BODIES

Dr. Rudolph Virchow was perhaps the greatest physician of the nineteenth century. He lived during the Enlightenment and there were many scientific advances in all fields of knowledge, especially medicine. Dr. Virchow's remarkable conclusion about disease was, "All disease results from the body's reaction to noxious stimuli." Genetic diseases were not known and most diseases were from infections at the time but considering genetic defects to produce noxious stimuli, Virchow's observation is broadly applicable. There is a tendency to consider illnesses' character to be determined by the cause (noxious stimuli) when the illness is from our own body's reactions. However, considering the noxious agent causes the reaction it remains causal but the importance in knowing the difference lies in prevention by avoiding the cause.

When we get poison ivy, it is easy to understand that a chemical from the leaves of a plant has come in contact with your skin causing it to become inflamed. The inflamed skin (Toxicodendron dermatitis is the "puffed-up" name for poison ivy) is the result of the exposed person's skin's acute reaction to a noxious stimulus, not the property of the chemical on the leaves.

Not convinced? People vary in their sensitivities to poison ivy. My neighbor contracted poison ivy requiring a doctor visit and steroid injections when weeding a shared flowerbed. I went out and completed the weeding gloveless without a blemish. People's bodily reactions constitute the disease and, when advanced, the illness.

There is a difference between the disease and the illness it produces. My neighbor with the painful rash suffered from the illness termed dermatitis (skin inflammation) caused by the disease. –itis denotes inflammation. Appendicitis is inflammation of the appendix. Chronic inflammation is a major cause of chronic (long-lasting) diseases and will be thoroughly discussed in a later chapter.

Getting back to Virchow's defining discovery, the derivative assumptions to avoid disease are clear. First, avoid noxious stimuli to prevent the body from reacting to them. The problem is that most harmful stimuli are unappreciated. Smoke from a bonfire is obviously noxious and everyone moves as the wind changes but once a smoker gets used to smoke from cigarettes the sensation is not seen as unpleasant but the smoke remains noxious to the body. Microscopic changes are visible in the lungs soon after a person starts to smoke.

Substantial overeating strains the liver, GI tract, and hormonal system, and overloads blood vessels with excess sugar, fats, and cholesterol causing the blood vessel lining to react by thickening and eventually forming plaque. These microscopic changes are also visible in young overeaters decades before illness.

Workers in plants where wood is prepared by treatment with coal tar have repeated skin exposure, which over two or three decades produces high rates of skin cancers because the substance is noxious to their skin. Their body's lengthy reactions to noxious substances brought about the cancers. There are large numbers of pollutant chemicals, solid particles, and biologicals known to harm humans which the government attempts to regulate. The US government has banned over 50 pesticides. These noxious substances are capable of inciting the body to develop a disease state.

Our amazing bodies are alert to protect us from the many dangers our environment poses. The body's defenses are poised to react when triggered. Sometimes this is an overreaction, causing more damage than had if the threat simply been allowed to run its course. In rare instances, people can be stung by a bee or eat something that is allergenic for them and even die. Again, it is their body's reaction, not the agent itself. These unfortunates with the sword of Damocles suspended by a thread overhead have extreme sensitivity to a foreign substance and must take precautions to avoid exposure.

Almost all of the chronic diseases are the result of years of inflammation that is mild enough to be unnoticed. Cancers of most organs are produced incrementally over decades including skin, lung, liver, breast, GI tract, and female genital tract. Chronic inflammation is operative in producing the vascular disease responsible for heart attacks and strokes.

Almost all of the complex functions of our body, digestion, respiration, metabolism, circulation, and countless other functions occur without our awareness; our bodies are on autopilot and react independently outside of our control. People with heart disease can inadvertently initiate a stress reaction making their diseased heart work hard enough to precipitate a heart attack. This sounds like an evolutionary design flaw until one looks at why the design got that way.

The release of stress hormones prepares the individual maximally for fight or flight. There are still situations when individuals under extreme duress perform superhuman tasks. These feats are possible from chemical reactions of the stress hormones. Prehistory of humanity's prehistoric survival depended on the ability to compete in an extremely dangerous environment; the best stress reactors had a survival advantage. Survival mechanisms such as the "stress reaction" persist into old age even though dangers from wild animals have ceased long ago. John Hunter, the most famous physician of his time, discoverer of the circulation, suffered terribly from the combination of anger and heart disease–caused angina. He was accustomed to say, "My life is in the hands of any rascal who chooses to annoy and tease me." He died in 1793 after an argument.

Thus, the body's reactions are the primary cause of most illnesses after disease has set the stage. It is important to prepare your body to react favorably in situations that could threaten your health. The core of preventative medicine is to arrange healthful behaviors and the physician is not in charge, the body's owner is responsible. In the following chapters methods to prepare your body to react favorably will be discussed in detail.

HOW TO DEAL WITH CHRONIC DISEASE: KNOW YOUR ENEMY

Upon diagnosis with a chronic disease, expend the effort to become acquainted with its nature. Behaviors can be changed to lessen the illness it causes; after all, it will be your companion for a long time. Become an expert on the chronic diseases you have to live with and those you want to avoid. Understand how the disease causes illness and the basic mechanism of the treatment. If a disease has fluctuations in the severity of the illness, keep a log detailing the circumstances of occurrence, what actions worsened or bettered symptoms. In other words, study your particular disease.

Your doctor knows the generalities of your disease but you know the specifics. My personal physician is recognized as being at the top of his specialty. He prescribed a new medication and I developed annoying tingling. He had never had a patient develop tingling from that medicine and did not consider that the medication caused it. I stopped the medicine and the tingling stopped. I restarted it and, Eureka, tingling. Medicine is complex beyond belief because biology is so variable.

Bodies experience considerable wear to keep us alive. The lining of the upper gastrointestinal tract is replaced every 48 hours. After all, the lining cells are exposed to acids and enzymes that dismantle ingested cells from plants and animals. It is amazing in such an environment that gastrointestinal disease is not more common. Our body's regenerative power depends on whether we maintain beneficial habits.

Our hearts beat approximately over one hundred thousand times each day producing a pulse with an associated shear force on vascular walls throughout the body. One can feel the force expanding the vascular walls when taking a pulse. Our heart and other vessels can be exposed to noxious stimuli from a number of sources. Tobacco toxins, air pollutants, injury from pounding of high blood pressure, high cholesterol, and others we don't yet appreciate. The metabolic disturbance of healing diabetes adds to the other reactions. Our body's regenerative power depends on limiting noxious stimuli.

Injuries require healing and the healing process when acute replaces the damaged tissue with scar, just as one sees on the skin that is acute healing. Chronic healing is more of a repeated irritation that produces an inflammation with local biochemical changes without scar. Unlike poison ivy where the immediate reaction clearly identifies the causative agent, agents injuring blood vessels and causing cancer have latent periods of decades before illness erupts. The changed biochemical milieu gradually results in plaque buildup in arteries or notable differences in cells as a precancerous state. Then the probability of illness increases steadily with continued exposure. The probability of lung cancer from smoking increases steadily depending on the number of years one smokes and the amount consumed.

It is easy to overlook the cause of a deleterious result if it takes a long time to become noticeable. Most of the diseases that kill are from exposure to agents that mildly injure or factors that increase susceptibility to noxious stimuli. Smoking does not appreciably increase lung cancer until one has smoked 20 years. The injury in chronic diseases is termed "subclinical," which means the injury does not produce symptoms that signal it is harmful.

Most of the dreaded chronic diseases are identifiable microscopically years before manifesting as illness and being diagnosed. There are many conditions that are likely to become cancerous—termed "precancerous" (pre = before, cancerous = producing cancer). In other words, they are settings where tissue changes can be identified that are not yet cancerous but in time are likely to worsen into cancers. Lesions that in their present state are not harmful but as they worsen over time will become so, strongly indicating that most of the bad diseases are preventable if our bodies can slow their progression. Included among those routinely monitored by testing are skin, cervix, and colon. Finding these threatening cellular changes and removing them early is lifesaving.

Other areas recognized to have long-standing tissue changes preceding overt cancer include: esophagus, stomach, thyroid, lung, pancreas, and liver. From the wide diversity of organs affected, one can assume that cancers everywhere develop slowly and are overt when they get out of control. An amazingly high number of older men have prostate cancer that never develops symptoms or causes problems. This fact is known from sections of the prostate glands of men at autopsy who died of other causes.

In some instances, the noxious agent impairs the body's ability to make repairs from normal wear and tear. In other instances, the body's inflammatory system continues to work overtime resulting in pain and deformity such as in arthritis. Steroids and other anti-inflammatory medicines work by shutting down the bodies' ability to generate the inflammatory response but also reduce the mechanism for making repairs.

There are limited numbers of ways to remove substances from the body because excretions are limited. Excretions include feces, urine, sweat, and in the case of volatile substances by breathing. Mechanisms are in place to maintain equilibrium within close parameters, especially chemical compositions. If one drinks excess water, within minutes the kidneys increase urine output. Kidneys are the first line of defense but they can only deal with water-soluble substances that are small molecules. The liver is the second line of defense. It detoxifies thousands of potentially harmful substances and excretes them in bile, which exits in feces.

Certain substances are not easily eliminated and accumulate. Included are many so-called toxic waste substances from industrial pollution and banned pesticides. Governmental regulatory agencies are all that stands between us and those who pollute and they don't do a good job. Contamination of waterways and airways with hazardous substances is very dangerous long-term to wildlife and humans. Fish and other creatures reach high tissue levels over time and when eaten can cause human disease. Considering the insidious danger not to the environment per se but to life in the environment, perhaps even more should be done by the Environmental Protection Agency (EPA) in this regard.

Heavy metals also accumulate imperceptibly. The phrase "mad as a hatter" has an interesting origin. When beaver hats were popular, they were hand-made and mercury was used in their manufacture. As the hatters worked the mercury into the material, minute amounts were absorbed through their skin. When enough had accumulated, hatters developed noticeable tremors and became irrational—ergo, they became "mad hatters." Reliable organizations such as Consumer Reports advise limiting tuna consumption, especially in children, because of the mercury content.

Asbestos is a mineral with valuable properties as a shield against heat used to retard fire. It was useful in ships, buildings, and in any construction where spread of fire would be a problem. Unfortunately, minute particles accumulate in the lungs and half a lifetime later cause a particularly bad cancer—mesothelioma.

Disease can result from a lack of essential substances, not just an excess. Everyone knows that water deficiency results in dehydration. Dehydration is considered causal to a number of diseases but not a disease in itself. Vitamins are good examples of substances whose lack causes disease. The term "vit-amin" originally meant vital amines. Vitamins are substances that are essential to our metabolism that our bodies do not manufacture in sufficient quantities. They must be taken in our diets.

Substances that are taken into the body in small amounts over long periods of time and accumulate injury are potentially harmful. Tobacco smoke is such a substance, even in the diluted form of second-hand smoke.

Energy from sun or X-rays gradually damages skin DNA, causing aging and if severe enough skin cancer. It is an unfortunate side effect because before sunlight was known to be harmful, the tan color it induced exuded health and vitality. Additionally, tanning produces vitamin D and other substances that can cause a feeling of well-being. Skin damage from sun exposure and genetic alterations from X-ray studies accumulate over a lifetime and are not reversible. Not so with tobacco residue; stopping smoking, the increased risk of a heart attack reverts rapidly and the cancer risk returns to normal over time.

Diseases can cause illnesses, rapidly or slowly; otherwise they would be unimportant. As Gertrude Stein summed, "To be a difference, it has to make a difference." Diseases may or may not cause illnesses. Prostate cancer that does not cause illness or that the illness is unappreciated is common in elderly men.

Chronic diseases are present for decades before surfacing as illnesses. A certain degree of disease severity must develop before producing illness. Autopsies in elderly men reveal a surprising incidence of prostate cancer that because of its slow growth never produced illness and was of no consequence even though nests of tumor cells had been there for decades. Most of the chronic diseases are eventually not so benign but they have been developing for decades. They are of no consequence as long as they don't exceed the ability of the body to control them.

Some chronic diseases are so prevalent past middle age that they are considered an inevitable part of aging. This statement is not true. Chronic disease before and after harming is the sum of little injuries that accumulate. While most that age have chronic disease, which takes a long time to harm, it can be slowed or even reversed by attention to healthy lifestyles. The most important takeaway lesson from this book is that chronic diseases are potential disasters which mostly can be dealt with or avoided by choices.

A good example of prevention of harm is the wearing of seatbelts. When the emergency room receives notification that an injured patient is being brought in, the utmost indicator that their injuries are severe is "ejected from vehicle." That means they were not seat-belted. Three-fourths will die. Get with the prevention program.

Chapter 4

What Keeps You Alive?
The Miracle of Metabolism

WHAT IS METABOLISM?

In the classic movie *City Slickers*, Curley, the trail boss, said it all: "When it comes to life, there is just one thing" and he was correct. All living things, including humans, are alive because of the mystical magic of metabolism. You are as healthy and as youthful as your metabolism. As we age, we blame weight gain on our metabolism, which is correct but our metabolism is much more important than the regulation of our weight. As in all things, nothing is inevitable. You can even avoid taxes—if you get elected to congress. Seriously, you can alter your metabolism. It is yet another example of mistakes in taking important things for granted.

The cells of our bodies are more numerous on average than the national debt—30 trillion! Metabolism sums the trillions upon trillions of dynamic biochemical reactions continuously taking place every second to keep our bodies functioning—staying alive and healthy. These incredible reactions convert food into energy and other necessary substances allowing life. Cars take us where we want to go because thousands of parts function coherently and our bodies are alive because these countless coherent biochemical reactions make it so.

Although medical science is remarkable and includes the greatest brainpower on the planet, scientists *discover new biochemical reactions every day*. Metabolism need not be a scary, complicated, seemingly undefinable subject. Using broad strokes, it is very understandable and helpful in making wise lifestyle decisions. You don't have to be overwhelmed by all of this; the forest of metabolism that you need to know about is straightforward; the trees that the scientists study are complex.

Football is a good metaphor for this situation; a playbook has dozens of complex diagrams about what 11 players should do when an individual play is called. Nevertheless, simply knowing the fact that the team carrying the football across the opposing team's goalposts most wins is adequate to understanding the game, without which the activity does not make much sense.

Living matter, us included, makes up an extremely small part of the known universe; living matter is exceedingly special. If the combined weight of living material (biomass) on Earth equaled a penny (actually 500 billion tons), the nonliving mass of our solar system would equal a thousand trillion times our national debt. WOW! Thank goodness good things can come in small packages.

All these sophisticated life-sustaining processes are divisible into two types of reactions. The first type involved breaking down large molecules into smaller ones (catabolism), thereby producing nutrients for energy or obtaining essential building blocks for future assembly. The second set of reactions is combining the disassembled small molecules to assemble larger ones (anabolism) that are species-specific.

A good friend collects antique cars. In fact, he drives one. To get unavailable parts, they must be disassembled from other cars of the same model and reassembled, just as our body does with foodstuffs. Living plants create new building blocks, animals don't; animals use plant material to form their bodies. Also, predatory animals, such as humans (we are the most predatory creatures on the planet), use building blocks from both plants and other animals.

These disassembling and assembling activities include many complex steps that biochemists and molecular biologists spend their careers gradually unraveling. However, it is not necessary to know the steps to understand the process.

In most life-giving health-promoting processes, grasping the big picture is most important; it is the forest approach. As mentioned, the tree approach is what the biochemist scientists use when they study individual chemicals and their actions. The forest approach is much simpler; it allows nonscientists to understand precisely the important developments going on in our bodies.

Most molecular disassembling takes place in the intestinal tract and assembling takes place in the liver; these are the factories, the "General Motors" of our bodies. Each cell also has lesser abilities, such as auto repair facilities. However, when nutrients are unavailable as in starvation, the bodies' own tissues are in danger of becoming disassembled. The real problem with starvation is that the body disassembles important necessary molecules as well as unimportant ones. This is especially important in people who don't have extra essential molecules handy, as in the elderly.

WHAT ARE THE BASIC BUILDING BLOCKS OF METABOLISM?

Carbon and oxygen and are the keys to life as we know it. Carbon atoms provide the central framework, like Tinker Toy spools, allowing the complex molecules to form the blocks of life. Hydrogen, oxygen, nitrogen, and other atoms are arranged in unbelievably complex molecules with the central carbon spools.

Oxygen furnishes the necessary energy to build the structures of life. Scientists seeking planets suspected of harboring life forms examine the newly discovered planet's atmosphere for oxygen. Oxygen is the third most common element in the universe and the second most common element on the surface of Earth. Oxygen is very reactive chemically; it combines readily with other elements during oxygenation; it is a Bolshevik molecule—attacking other molecules. Forrest fires, internal combustion engines, rust, and animal cellular energy generation all result from oxygen combining with other atoms (called oxygenation). The chemical processes involving oxygen, releases energy, which is channeled into useful functions fuels life and is directly from our cells "burning" oxygen.

The energy rating of gasoline is in octanes, whereas our food, which is in fact our fuel, has its energy-producing level in calories, as everyone knows. A calorie is the heat energy to raise the temperature of a liter (a little less than a quart, 0.95 quart) of water one degree (Celsius)—not a lot of energy. Perhaps that is why we need several thousand calories a day.

Oxygenation resulting in fire is combustion, whereas the process in animal tissue is far more controlled by multiple chemical steps and is termed "respiration." Glucose is the principal fuel because it is readily accessible. Besides being made available with diet, glucose resides in storage tanks in the liver and skeletal muscle—ready on a minute-by-minute basis to be released.

THE PROCESS OF LIVING IS WHAT CAUSES AGING

When released, glucose as fuel must have an escort to open cellular doors so it can enter cells to provide energy. The escort is insulin, without which the released glucose accumulates in the bloodstream and the resulting disease is diabetes. In nondiabetics as much insulin is secreted as necessary to keep the blood glucose at acceptable levels. This means consuming more sugar floors the metabolic gas pedal, making the furnaces run faster, and increases the harmful sparks. Sweetened sodas are among the worst for making cells rev up and cause more damage, thus aging our cells faster.[1]

The total amount of glucose consumed is important for damage to occur but another consideration applies: the rate at which sugar is absorbed from foodstuffs because different foods have different rates of absorption of sugars they contain. The fastest rate—that is, the most harmful absorption—is pure sugar. This is why food products that add extra sugar are particularly bad for your metabolism and, thus, bad for your body. The rate sugar is absorbed from various foodstuffs is important; it is called the glycemic index of food. It takes time for the digestive process to release sugar from beans, most fruits (excluding watermelon), and vegetables. So, the amount of sugar and rate it is absorbed are important to your cellular health. Imagine a coal-burning furnace with a pile of coal to be burned. The heat produced would depend on the size of the pile and the rate the attendant shoveled the coal into the furnace. The faster the absorption is, the hotter the fire and greater the damage. Eureka.

Within each cell are tiny furnaces—called mitochondria—where oxygen from the bloodstream combines with fuel from food, mainly sugars, in a series of controlled chemical reactions. These microscopic furnaces, as efficient as they are, still toss off sparks just as a campfire would. The sparks, called free radicals, are unstable extremist molecules that need to attach and interact with other molecules.

Free radicals are not selective; any molecule will do. They mostly land on nonessential molecules but since they change the chemical structure of molecules with which they interact they occasionally alter important molecules. This alteration is very important because the molecular structure determines what the molecule does. The many molecules in cells function very specifically and small changes drastically alter their function, especially DNA segments. General molecular structure determines whether molecules function as coffee cups or computers.

Accumulated damage leads to aging-associated degenerative diseases because disease is from insufficient ability of our bodies to function. It is if a business that depends on its employees who function to provide services had a large number come down with the flu. Moreover, not just diseases, free radical damage actually is responsible for aging; if there were no free radicals, all living organisms would remain forever pristine. Of course, they would not be alive because the life force requires that sparks be produced.

The unbalanced metabolic rate determines our fate. Our metabolism produces free radicals and they must be balanced with antioxidants to lessen damage, which occurs because antioxidants neutralize free radicals. Our total un-neutralized sparks increases the rate of cellular damage; this is termed "oxidative stress."

The energy intake from food is similar to stoking the firebox where larger amounts of coal produces increased fire, which produces more sparks, or, in the body, increased free radicals. This explains why creatures with higher energy intakes age faster; they produce more damaging free radicals.

Machines that run faster and longer wear out sooner. Machines that run faster that are not maintained with proper lubrication wear out even faster. It appears similar in animals that have higher metabolic rates and have shorter lifespans.[2] Hummingbirds live only a few years with many dying in less than a year. Houseflies live less than a month and their lifespan can be closely predicted by oxidative damage from free radical "sparks."[3] All living creatures have the same metabolism associated problems, not just humans.

The antidote for free radicals, since free radicals are oxidants (substances produced by the fire of metabolism called oxidation), is antioxidants. Antioxidants are tiny spark (free radical) extinguishers. Antioxidants attach to the free radicals before they can damage cells and then the inert molecule produced is disposed of in the urine; a neat system to be sure. Life exists beyond all odds against it and like someone noted, "What does exist can exist." Amen.

Antioxidants are either ingested or produced by the body. The more antioxidants you contain, the more slowly you age. Fruits, vegetables, beans, olive oil, and nuts have higher concentrations of health-promoting antioxidants. They certainly are the elements responsible for the wholesome effects of the Mediterranean diet. The body produces antioxidants as well—more than we absorb in our diet. Exercise produces the need for more energy expenditure; so, the fires burn more intensely. Instead of producing more free radical damage, exercise reduces the damage and wear of free radicals by over-producing antioxidants.

The body has developed protective mechanisms against damage from bodily functions; otherwise, we would all die young. The challenge of exercise to the body by producing more free radical sparks, enhances the body's production of antioxidant fire extinguishers. It is similar to having larger, better-trained squads of first responders. And it is likely that this enhanced production of beneficial molecules works whenever needed, not just when you exercise.

Nutrients that emit the mainstream of the body's energy are sugars and fats. Proteins are the bricks and mortar of the body's material. The actual building blocks of protein are amino acids, which can be converted to energy when overabundant or necessary because other sources are lacking. Only 10% to 15% of the body's total energy is from protein, and energy from protein consumes 30% of its caloric content to convert amino acids into energy.

Fat is simpler to consume and takes one-tenth as much energy to process. Further, fat is high octane with nine calories per gram and by contrast protein and sugars have four calories per gram. Because of energy lost in conversion, the net caloric value of protein is 2.6 calories per gram. For reference, a nickel by law weighs 5 grams.

WHY DO WE PREFER CERTAIN FOODS

Fatty foods are universally preferred. Fatty foods taste better, because we are programed that way; they have a smoother more satisfying mouth feel, and are delightfully crispy when fried. Universal behaviors are not normally cultural as cultures vary; universal behaviors are likely to have genetic origins. Prehistorical cultures would have experienced unpredictable food supplies and needed to expend considerable energy in hunting and gathering. They, also, lacked methods of preservation, so, eating habits would have been opportunistic.

Their insurance against starvation would have been to consume the most calories when food was available which would be from fatty meals. Evolution works by who survives to pass on genes and those consuming more calories would have had a better chance of not starving. But why should the preference for high caloric foods persist for millennia after the development of agriculture and animal husbandry made it unnecessary? Its persistence is especially interesting because of the widespread knowledge that a diet of high caloric foods is unhealthy.

Evolutionary survival trends, once established, persist until they become detrimental to a population before mating age. Just like paraphrasing the Las Vegas saying: What evolution does stays in evolution. For example, bodily speed and hand–eye coordination were important for success in hunting and warfare but have been replaced by technology. Nevertheless, almost all modern sports emphasize one or both of these skills. We celebrate pitchers, quarterbacks, and point guards. We are much more than we eat but our bodies are composed of what we eat. It is important, as has been discussed, that we consume varied healthy diets to promote good health.

One of the most important aspects of metabolism is our basal metabolic rate, which is the rate of energy consumption required to keep our body alive. Considering just "keepin alive" consumption requires over 60% of our caloric intake.

Tissues vary in the caloric requirements to stay alive. Fat cells require very little energy to keep alive (13 calories/pound/day); fat cells are like warehouses. But muscle is more like Grand Central Station having increased activity and thus requiring a larger amount (60 calories/pound/day) to stay alive. Without increased activity, we steadily lose muscle which (admit it) is replaced by fat.

Replacement of ten pounds of muscle by fat reduces our energy consumption by a big mac a day, which, if caloric intake remains the same, can cause the gain of a pound a week!

WATER IS IMPORTANT

Water is the molecular highway that allows metabolism to take place. All of the transport of the molecules of life and their interactions occur in water. Life itself began in water. The metaphorical Biblical phrase "Living Water" is biologically correct. Sixty percent of the human body is water. To remain healthy, one must be well hydrated.

Years ago when I was an intern at the once famous but now closed Philadelphia General Hospital, elderly patients residing at a huge nursing home would become severely dehydrated and lapse into coma with very low blood pressure. In the ER we would start an IV, run in fluid, and they would soon awaken. The local-jargon diagnosis was "instant people syndrome."

Consider the numerous ways water is lost from our bodies: obvious losses include excretions such as sweat, saliva, urine, and bowel movements. Then there are the irregular losses from vomiting or diarrhea. Less appreciated are what medicine terms "insensible losses" or "invisible losses." Blowing one's breath on a window pane, especially a cold one will cause it to fog up from condensation of water vapor. We exhale water vapor with every breath, exhaling over a pint of water every day. Water continually evaporates from our skin without the formation of droplets of sweat. In average sized individuals, these unappreciated losses total almost four 8-ounce glasses of water a day.

The elderly are particularly vulnerable to dehydration.[4] Those over 65 years have decreased renal function, are often taking multiple medications, and their sensation of thirst is reduced. In a large German study, 28% of subjects 65–75 years and 41% of those over 85 years did not meet daily water intake recommendations.[5]

There are a number of infirmities resulting from dehydration: decreased mental functioning, tiredness, lethargy, and cramps can occur. More seriously, dehydration predisposes to blood clots forming in blood vessels. Illnesses especially with GI losses or fever can increase to need for more fluid consumption and care must be taken to avoid dehydration.

Dehydration's signs can be subtle but awareness is important. First, a dry mouth and thirst signs are primary. Marked reduction in the amount of urine produced and the urine may appear slightly darker. The skin is dry and when pulled on does not snap right back. Normally there is a slight moisture in the armpit regions. When any of these signs are present water intake should be increased.

The secret of life is "How much is enough?" A quart of total fluid intake (four 8-ounce cups/day) for every 50 pounds of body weight is a good rule of thumb. That amount includes beverages, water, and the fluids in food. Normally, a little over a cup of water is produced daily from food consumption. Coffee, tea, and alcohol contain diuretics and cause more urine to be formed so they contribute to intake less than the amount consumed. It is estimated that water in food supplies and water produced by metabolism contribute 20% of our intake. Using the previous formula (four 8-ounce glasses of fluid/50 pounds body weight) and subtracting 20% a 150-pound person should consume ten 8-ounce glasses of fluid, including beverages, daily. The Institute of Medicine recommends more (13 cups for men and 9 for women). However, I do not find their recommendation supported by data. Consumption of fluid should be in small amounts spread over the day, not in few large volumes, such as chugging a bottle of water, because the resulting increase in urine output will negate the benefit.

DIGESTION MADE SIMPLE: YOU ARE WHAT YOU EAT

Food consumption supplies nutrients that are the body's fuel and building materials. Aside from minerals, big-molecule nutrients useful to animals are the tissues of other living creatures that also are species-specific and must be disassembled into basic building blocks and absorbed.

These elemental nutritional fragments are amino acids, simple sugars, and fatty acids. Disassembling macromolecules takes place in the gastrointestinal tract starting with the chewing of food and mixing it with saliva and continues until the residual is expelled as feces. The disassembling starts in your mouth with sugars. Chew bread for a few minutes and it will become sweet as the sugar is released from enzymes contained in saliva. The digestive process starts in the mouth.

However, the frontline responsible tissues for digestion are principally the lining of the small intestines, pancreas, and the liver. Assembling the building blocks produced by breaking down nutrients is done inside the cells. Liver cells are assemblage factories making most of the widely distributed proteins and detoxifying potentially harmful substances such as drugs and alcohol, which is why alcohol in excess damages the liver. Just as the heart is the center of the circulation, the liver is the center of metabolism.

Broadly, nutrient processing can be considered to consist of three phases: absorption, processing, and elimination. The overall absorption of nutrients is termed "digestion." Digestion is a very efficient process but there is an important point that should be obvious but must be stressed: digestion can only offer the body nutrients that can be broken down from foods that are eaten. In marked contrast to plants, animal bodies, especially the complex higher animal bodies, do not manufacture their life substance from scratch; the molecules composing animal tissues and organs are reassembled from plant and other animal tissues. This means that what humans consume is vital to supply the body's needs.

Human bodies need to consume thirteen vitamins, two essential fatty acids (from fat), eight essential amino acids (from protein), and sixteen necessary minerals.

The least amount of various nutrients that are needed is written on packaged foods as minimum daily requirements. In general, varied diets will adequately supply the minimum daily requirements of essential nutrients. Moderation and diversification such as in the stock market is for the most part the secret of a healthy diet. Foods differ in the building blocks and minerals they contain and variation of consumption is necessary.

Before the last century, sailor's diets on long journeys consisted of cured meats and grain because fruits and vegetables would spoil. Absence of vitamin C caused the dreadful disease known as scurvy. James Lind, a surgeon in the British Navy, discovered that scurvy could be avoided by eating citrus fruit in 1753. British sailors became known as Limeys because they were given lime juice on long voyages.

Currently, the public concept of dietary health regarding vitamins is that more is better. More in biology is not always better. Vitamins and minerals can be taken in excess and produce illness instead of being more healthy. Vitamins broadly are of two types: water-soluble and fat-soluble. Nine vitamins can be dissolved in water and four vitamins dissolve in fats. When excess, unneeded water-soluble vitamins are ingested, they are eliminated in urine, so water-soluble vitamins have a safety net—the kidneys. The fat-soluble vitamins cannot be urinated away; they must be metabolized and besides they accumulate in fatty body tissues. Toxic levels produce diseases termed hyper-vitamin-oses. Remember –oses designate diseases not caused by infections. Fat-soluble vitamins can be remembered by the phrase "Eek watch out for the DEAK," meaning vitamins D, E, A, and K must be taken in guarded amounts. Vitamin D is sometimes the exception; even in varied diets vitamin D may be deficient, especially in the elderly.

Minerals also can be taken in excess. There are at least 16 necessary minerals in the human body. Seven are the major minerals and nine are termed "trace" minerals because of their small amounts. Among the major minerals (called electrolytes in medicine because they have electrical charges) seven are regularly measured by blood tests. Minerals, except for heavy metals, are easily eliminated by the kidneys which have exquisitely sensitive processes to keep the concentrations within narrow limits.

People with kidney disease must be careful about mineral intake. The major minerals are healthy only within narrow limits. Our bodies are extremely well engineered. Potassium may be lost in excess when taking water pills and extra should be taken or heart rhythms can become abnormal. Contrarily, potassium in excess makes the heart stop. Potassium is the electrolyte injected for executions but is essential for life in the right amounts. Wow! Don't become excessively concerned; if your kidneys are not diseased, there is almost no chance your potassium consumption can endanger your life.

Health is optimized by sufficient intake of these simple substances of life, which besides water, as mentioned, includes electrolytes, generally referred to as salts. There are four key electrolytes: sodium (in common table salt), calcium residing in bones, potassium residing in cells, and magnesium.

Almost a half century ago a landmark study was done in the isolated Cook Islands located in the South Pacific. The islands comprise 93 square miles located in ocean area larger than Alaska. The capital island has had trade with international shipping for centuries and has a "western" diet. Their diet was compared with an isolated island without "western" influence. The average salt intake was significantly higher on the westernized island where, just as in western locales, blood pressure rose steadily as people aged. The isolated island imported no table salt. In marked contrast, on the isolated salt-restricted island blood pressure remained low as natives aged into the 70s.[6]

Magnesium is the fourth most prevalent electrolyte in human bodies and the only one that is not adequately supplied by many diets. American diets are often inadequate to prevent chronic magnesium deficiencies.[7] Overall one-fourth of diets are insufficient in magnesium and this deficient intake increases to 80% in the elderly. Magnesium is added by eating a variety of nuts, seeds, herbs, and grains that may not be commonly included in American diets: Brazil nuts, molasses, rice, and dark chocolate are examples of foods rich in magnesium.

Magnesium is not commonly ordered in laboratory tests as are three other electrolytes (sodium, potassium, and calcium). Magnesium is necessary for optimal functioning of over three hundred essential biochemical reactions. It promotes muscle, nerve, and bone health. Magnesium stabilizes the heart rhythm, provides reactions for a healthy immune system, and keeps bone tissue strong. Deficiencies have been linked to cardiovascular disease, high blood pressure, diabetes, sudden death syndrome, migraine headaches, and increased colon cancer. Further, higher intake of magnesium has been shown to reduce colon and rectal cancer.[8]

Magnesium excretion is increased when taking diuretics or drinking alcohol. One or two 400 mg capsules of magnesium oxide daily will supply adequate amounts. When first starting supplementation, loose stools may occur, so it is best to take the capsules in the morning with breakfast. After all milk of magnesia is a laxative. Switching to magnesium aspartate is tolerated better in some people. Loose stools usually stop with time as the body becomes used to an increased intake.

Controlling metabolism is the best way to control weight. The key measurement is the basal metabolic rate (BMR, the amount of calories the body requires at rest). The BMR consumption varies most with the pounds of muscle the body has. Muscle loss begins after age 25 and averages about 0.5% annually. For every 10 pounds of muscle lost 600 less calories are needed daily but our appetites do not correspondingly decrease. Muscle loss reversal is possible with exercise and especially by moderate weight training. In multiple studies, short-term weight training in elderly men, even men over 80 years, resulted in significant gains in strength and muscle mass.

Simple dietary changes that become enjoyable can improve metabolism. Besides containing far fewer calories than fat, protein has other weight control advantages. Consuming excess protein does not produce fat for storage nearly as easily as fat or sugar. Foods with ample protein are more filling. And it is well known by nutritionists that protein consumption temporarily speeds up overall metabolism producing heat and consuming calories. This acceleration of metabolism is specific to protein—termed "specific dynamic action." After meals, protein intake increases metabolism by 25% for a few hours. Fat tends to slow metabolism, which is why everyone sits around in a listless state or falls asleep watching television.

Next, there are effective measures to limit caloric intake. Portion control is an easier less cumbersome method than calorie counting. Okinawans eat until they are 80% full, not stuffed. Instead of a blessing before meals, they say eat until 80% full. They are the longest-lived group on the planet. When eating out, stop when satisfied and take the remainder home or split an order; and although it is said there is none, it provides a FREE LUNCH. After all, we were trained from early childhood to "clean our plates." Most restaurants seek to keep business with generous portions. Don't regress to childhood behaviors; exploit this by splitting and "takee outee." You will truly enjoy that less becomes more. At home, use small plates and eat slowly savoring each bite. You will soon begin to see results and will generate less free radicals. You are aging slower with each meal.

Chapter 5

Inflammation

The Crucible of Age-Related Disease

WHAT IS INFLAMMATION'S ROLE IN HEALTH?

As mentioned, in acute (rapidly developing) diseases such as infections, a specific bacterium or virus is usually readily identifiable. It is much harder, however, for scientific inquiry to determine the basic cause of age-related (slowly developing) diseases. Take heart disease, for instance: the higher your "bad" cholesterol (LDL), the greater your risk of heart attack or stroke. That makes high cholesterol a risk factor—it increases the likelihood that disease will develop faster in the arteries—but it is not factually a cause of heart attacks. Generally, age-related disease is the same as lifestyle-related disease, which assigns responsibility.

Age-related diseases—heart disease, diabetes, cancer, chronic obstructive pulmonary disease, obesity—develop slowly because that is their nature, which is exactly why chronic diseases become more common as we age. It is because the damage leading to illnesses accumulates slowly.

Many people assume, therefore, that the processes of aging and development of a chronic disease are the same, or correlated as parallel phenomena. And this is partly true but the real truth is this: continuing inflammation is what accelerates the rate of aging, but more important the onset or worsening of age-related (chronic) disease—not purely the passage of time. Aging is an independent biochemical process, differing from the processes causing our bodies to become suddenly impaired from illnesses. And what is this avoidable root cause of impairment of our health?

Recently, the National Institutes of Health, arguably the most influential medical body in the world, hosted a conference on the inflammation of aging (termed "inflammaging"). At the conference, it noted that "most, if not all, age-related diseases share an inflammatory pathogenesis" or root cause. It turns out that ongoing inflammation is the crux of the diseases of advancing age, the common denominator, you could say. Understanding this connection means we have a chance at slowing the aging process as well as avoiding aging-related diseases.

Every elderly person (and many younger ones) has undeniable evidence of chronic disease, which can also be viewed simply as biological corrosion. The first signs—mostly microscopic—can be stabilized, or allowed to eventually override the body's ability to prevent symptoms. Symptoms are the clarion call of illnesses. Evidence of inflammation predicts the pace of advance of a chronic disease to the point of illness.

Medical research on the cause of physical decline and diseases of aging can study only small, rather limited questions. It must be a "trees" rather than "forest" focus because the human body is too complex to study in detail overall. The bits and pieces are often well understood but how they fit together is not. Imagine a huge factory where thousands of steps are required to manufacture a car. One group on the assembly line installs the dashboard, becoming efficient at attaching the right screws and welds to do the job. Dozens of other groups install the gauges, or radios, or glove compartments. Each group is expert at one small component of the end product: an automobile. Scientists studying the human body look at specific areas because the overall picture is just too complex. They are medical experts with deep knowledge of a narrow segment of human life.

Medical knowledge, therefore, advances in fits and starts, mostly by assembling pieces of the puzzle over time and with much effort. Because age-related diseases now are responsible for 70% of all deaths, 92% of deaths in the elderly, and 99% of suffering, a great deal of research has been focused on them. The findings point to a common thread: low-grade continuing inflammation. Inflammation is the purpose of the immune system.

What Is the Immune System?

Our bodies have a multitude of "systems" that keep us alive and functioning, named according to the major task performed—the nervous system, digestive system, cardiovascular system, and so on—but the system with the most important role in our overall adult health is the immune system—overall is the key concept.

The immune system recognizes injury at the cellular level and sets off early alarms for prevention of further damage, initiating cleanup and repair. Its primary function is to protect against acute disease, so how can it be implicated in aging-associated disease?

Evolution designed the immune system to eliminate microscopic invaders (bacteria, viruses, fungi, and parasites), and to clean up damaged tissue, healing wounds from a variety of injuries. Its role was to protect us from the greatest dangers—infections and wounds—to help ensure survival of the species.

Age-associated diseases tend to occur after childrearing, in middle age and beyond, generally after a person has lived long enough to contribute offspring. Human's function is to carry and pass on genes. After sexual maturity, evolution doesn't care how long you live. The survival of the species has been safeguarded. As the matter of fact, older disabled primitive people would have been a burden on the tribe and it is generally rumored that in prehistory when the older could not keep up they were left to die.

In many illnesses, the strength of the immune system is the deciding factor of outcome. Here's how it works: White blood cells (leukocytes, leuko-white, cytes-cells) reside in the blood, lymph nodes, spleen, bone marrow, and tissues in general. There are several kinds of white blood cells; each has a unique microscopic appearance and a unique job.

The "foot-soldier" cells (neutrophils) rush in and engulf micro-invaders, literally digesting them. They are the heroes of the immune system in that during the process of ingesting and digesting bacteria and fungi, they die—sometimes producing pus if they die in sufficient numbers. Pus is also composed of normal cells killed in the process of eliminating invaders—friendly fire, if you will. This killing of neutrals near the microscopic battleground demonstrates the deadly toxins secreted by immune cells to eliminate other threatening live organisms.

Other cells (lymphocytes) can be considered the equivalent of immune system "artillery," firing off antibodies and other substances that kill invaders. These antibody artillery shells are toxic to specific invaders, similar to laser-guided-bombs. Then there are the "police force" cells (NK cells, think: Natural Killer) to eliminate abnormal body cells, such as tumor cells or cells infected with a virus. (This description of the role of the white blood cells is a simplification of a very complex system and there are a number of supportive systems that are essential but secondary.)

The lymphocytes are concentrated in bases, like garrisons of troops, and appropriately called lymph nodes. The circulatory system oozes fluid in the microscopic portion of the circulation from capillaries (between the arteries and veins) to convey nutrients. This escaped fluid is lymph and of enough volume that it must be returned to the body's blood stream. A network of ducts (lymphatics) that are separate from but usually accompany the blood vessels returns the overflow to the circulation. Unlike blood, lymph is usually clear or slightly cloudy, which probably accounts for its name; lymph derives from a Latin root meaning water.

The excess fluid released in the tissue returns to the blood by a separate series of vessels, the lymphatics, which carry lymph and go through the lymph nodes. Lymph nodes are located at key sites such as the groin for the legs and the armpits for the arms. When you have a sore throat, you may notice lumps in your neck; these are neck (cervical) lymph nodes gearing up to do their job. The lymph flow is another biological design marvel—the reclaimed lymph transports dangerous microorganisms from the tissues directly into the lymph nodes, which alerts the white blood cells to become active early. The lymph nodes, thus, serve as "military" checkpoints to increase protection from infection. They trap cancer, too.

Cancer cells lodge first in nodes that drain their locations fluid (regional nodes), delaying it from becoming widespread. This allows surgeons to remove more advanced cancers completely than would otherwise be possible if cancer cells went directly into the bloodstream. The extent to which cancer cells actively are killed by white blood cells located in lymph nodes is not well understood but we do know cancer cells are detained. Detaining them before they go everywhere is an important advantage, as mentioned, for surgical excision. Most cancer surgery removes lymph nodes where lymph from a cancer would drain and if there is no cancer found in the nodes, it is a favorable sign.

Although lymph nodes lie directly under the skin, they normally cannot be felt. If they are evident to the touch, something is wrong and a visit to the doctor is needed. Locations that are able to be felt are in the armpits, groin, and front of the neck.

So, you could say the immune system is the body's police force and army combined. It is more complex than can be imagined. It gives us protection (immunity) from the dangerous world of microorganisms. Our immune system has its own CIA that recognizes the millions and millions, perhaps billions, of identifying molecules of invaders, and it stockpiles weapons to deploy defenses rapidly when attacked in the future. This incredible memory accumulates identifiers of more potential threats than our National Security Agency. This is why immunizations work: they add identifiers for specific germs that alert the immune system without it having to experience an illness.

Our immune system has its own alarm system that mobilizes white blood cells to where the body needs them. Tissue cells, when distressed about possible danger, secrete substances that make white blood cells rapidly take up positions where they are needed (cytokines; cyto = cell, kines = mover). Some of the substances released upon the initiation and continuation of inflammation circulate to the entire body. When the threat is sufficiently large the release of these substances cause one to become ill.

What I've just described is the short-term (acute) response of the immune system to threats. Acute threats arise from infections and injuries of any kind: traumatic, thermal, and chemical. Sudden responses to these acute threats are well suited to short-term protective solutions. Longer-term microbiological threats such as some tuberculosis, which is resistant to drug therapy, are more lethal. But the most lethal threat in America is the sustained inflammatory response. Continual long-term release of toxins damages slightly but the damage accumulates, which is the deadly part.

The immune system is our first responder to injuries and healing from wounds. It is a good rapid deployment system but a poor long-term occupier. If infections occur in bones, for example, the immune system is relatively ineffective and illnesses can persist until the infected bone is removed. Moreover, the stimulus commanding the body to respond lasts as long as our tissues are being injured or exposed to a noxious substance.

How Does the Immune System Produce Inflammation?

When a microorganism enters the body, an alarm is rapidly signaled by various cells, especially white blood cells residing in the tissues and even in fat cells, by the release of warning proteins (cytokines). These alarms occur with threats to cells from any possible cause—not just microorganisms. Cells not getting enough oxygen are being stressed and are a trigger for release.

Incidentally, as one accumulates body fat, fat cells grow larger. Excessively large fat cells overproduce a certain warning cytokine, thereby giving a false alarm and producing a state of chronic low-grade inflammation, which is one reason why obesity is now considered a chronic disease. Here's what's going on with these fat cells: Oxygen diffuses from the capillaries to cells and the distance traveled is important; when cells enlarge beyond diffusion's ability to sustain them, they go into stages of suffocation and signal their damage. When released, these warning proteins dilate local small blood vessels and raise the local temperature but most of all attract more white cells. This initiates a well-coordinated complex response even though it's a false alarm. The problem: the response goes on and on. It is long-lasting, chronic.

It is important to realize that in addition to microorganism invasion, tissue injury from any cause can initiate inflammation. As Dr. Virchow noted in his famous maxim: "All disease is caused by the body's reaction to noxious stimuli." Microscopic invaders and wounds of any kind are noxious stimuli.

Bacteria, viruses, and other invaders can produce local inflammatory responses that become noticeable as whole-body responses once a certain threshold is reached. A minor scratch on the skin with minimal invasion causes local redness but you don't get sick the way you do when an abscess forms or you have the flu. With more serious infections, the inflammatory response is increased and the entire body responds by calling up the reserves, which causes a fever and a general "un-well" feeling. But the inflammatory response is never entirely local because the different potentially toxic substances (even if minimal) are diluted into the whole body. We do not consciously sense low-grade smoldering inflammation.

The immune system produces toxic substances to protect us against threats. These substances are generally contained but there is some spillover. Think of this dynamic as similar to a chemical plant that leaks a little pollution in the surrounding area. The harm may be imperceptible at first but its cumulative effect can cause long-term damage. In addition, the longer the chemical plant is in operation, the worse the harm. As we age, the immune system becomes less efficient. That means it loses some of its ability to protect us from acute disease and is less reliable. An older immune system is also activated more easily by false alarms and that's the most damaging aspect.

Sometimes, for reasons not well-understood, the immune system breaks down and begins to attack its own healthy cells, producing conditions called "autoimmune diseases." It is like having a military unit rebel, attacking its own government. There are more than 80 autoimmune diseases. Rheumatoid arthritis is a more common one. Fortunately, most of the more serious autoimmune diseases are not common. In an autoimmune disease, the mistaken response to a perceived threat is the threat. If not controlled, the falsely stimulated inflammatory process can damage and kill normal tissues.

In autoimmune diseases, something happens to cause the immune system to malfunction in a specific way. Rheumatoid arthritis, for example, affects the joints; sarcoidosis affects the lungs, primarily (other organs including the heart, esophagus, and skin may be affected as well); and so on. The prognosis for sarcoidosis depends on the level of cytokines; greater the levels of inflammation are associated with, the worse the long-term effects. In autoimmune cases, noxious stimuli that are unidentified, or something noxious produced by the body, causes the reactive disease.

Why does the immune system react mistakenly sometimes? Why does it not activate slower, perhaps, in stepwise fashion? The answer, perhaps, is similar to the stampeding of cattle when sudden stimuli, such as thunder and lightning, occur. Life in the wild (and in our bodies) is a zero-sum game. When the danger is real, the cattle who delay until they can decide whether the threat is serious will die because they will have given up their chance to escape. The immune system that delays sacrifices the best chance to survive because bacteria and other threats worsen with time.

The Evidence That Long-Standing Inflammation Causes Cancer

The noxious stimuli that produce cancers do not have to be noticeable—most often they are silent. The tarry oil creosote is used extensively to preserve wood. Workers exposed to creosote over many years develop skin cancer. Studies also show that long-term residents close to wood treatment plants have an increase in multiple chronic diseases.[1] The process whereby low-grade inflammation insidiously causes chronic diseases to worsen is clear; like biological systems, overall damage happens incrementally. This requires a latent period while the noxious agent gradually produces changes in the cells.

Remember that in the chapter on disease, Dr. Virchow's axiom mentioned was: "All disease is the bodies' reaction to a noxious agent." The noxious agent be it viruses, cigarette smoke, industrial pollutants, or our own bodies' misinterpretation of our cells as invaders continues to slowly damage cells. The period of time required is consistently about 20 years and as would be expected rates go higher, the more time elapses.

It is well known that some infections with viruses that persist and smolder cause cancer.[2] Currently, recommendations are for schoolchildren, especially girls, to be vaccinated against a sexually transmitted virus (HPV, human papilloma virus), which can cause cervical cancer in later life. Viruses causing hepatitis (C virus) result in liver cancer. Everyone knows that AIDS is bad.

Stomach ulcers and cancer (stomach cancer is particularly bad) have markedly decreased in the past several decades for a very simple reason. The stomach secretes acid about as strong as battery acid; thus, it was considered to be sterile, so no bacteria were looked for in the stomach. Big mistake. As it turned out, bacteria were causing stomach ulcers and stomach cancer because of increasing chronic inflammation.[3]

Other substances than cigarette smoke cause cancers of the lung; everyone knows from leg-biter law firm's television ads that past workers around asbestos get special forms of cancers in their chests. Asbestos causes cancer by being inhaled and the body cannot get rid of it. Asbestos causes a low-grade inflammatory response because of its noxious effect and the body responds with chronic inflammation.

There is a straightforward sense that prolonged irritation at a given site causes future problems we term "chronic disease" at that site. The messages about medicine's scientific discoveries that are presented to the public are at best simplistic. Sure localized incremental injury eventually produces problems locally but the damage is beyond local to be sure; the evidence of damage resulting in serious disease is widespread when inflammation is continuous for decades.

That smoking causes lung cancer seems straightforward; smoke contains cancer-causing agents (carcinogens). Nevertheless, ten cancers other than lung cancers double or more in smokers; female smokers have increased rates of cervical cancer; both sexes have increased bladder cancer. Those distant manifestations require deep inhales. No, this strongly suggests that local inflammation of the lung results in general detrimental effects. In fact, wherever the inflammation is localized can have effects on distant tissues. The distant effects depend on how severe an inflammatory response is produced. The lining of the lung if flattened would be about 160 square feet; this is about 30 times an average person's skin surface, which is a very large amount of inflammation.

A smoker's irritation of the airway's lining (bronchial epithelium) produces a local more pronounced inflammation (bronchitis) but there is measurable evidence of systemic inflammation as well. Smoke in our lungs—from cigarettes, cigars, or pipes—is actually generating widespread injury. Smokers are plagued with heart attacks and strokes; both diseases cause more deaths every year than smoking-related lung cancer.

Another challenging incisive situation is the connection of depressive disorders with chronic inflammation.[4] Many patients who are given treatment for hepatitis that stimulates their immune system and produces inflammation become clinically depressed. And "we cannot identify a single significant risk factor for MDD [Major Depressive Disorder], ranging from psychosocial stress and medical illness to obesity, diet, poverty, and sleep loss, that has not been repeatedly associated with increased inflammation."[4]

Another example of chronic inflammation underlying chronic disease is shown by the effects of aspirin. Aspirin decreases strokes and heart attacks because it decreases clotting but aspirin has also been shown to decrease cancer. All three of these maladies are chronic diseases. One large study showed that low-dose aspirin reduced the risk of dying from cancer.[5] Prostate cancer is reduced by long-standing aspirin use, in development of the disease and in less severe disease when it occurred.[6] Aspirin reduced esophageal,[7] colon, rectal,[8] and breast cancer.[9] There is controversy about breast cancer prevention but the National Institutes of Health-AARP Diet and Health Study surveyed over 127,000 women and found moderate benefit.[10]

These diseases have different pathological origins, different anatomical locations, and markedly dissimilar treatments. Yet, one medication's action reduces them all. The only possible mechanism is that there is a common root cause that aspirin mostly neutralizes: It is inflammation.

All of the common chronic diseases (even dementia) have a shared root: chronic persistent inflammation. Understanding that there is a direct association but a differing mechanism between long-term inflammation and aging allows us to build a plan for healthier aging. Their association stems from the fact that both occur over time. Different parts of your car wear over time but in differing ways. The engine wears from friction of motion, whereas the outside paint corrodes from weather.

Acute inflammation saves our lives; prolonged inflammation slowly causes damage; if allowed to continue, it kills us. Harmful bacteria living on the skin and in the bowel are deadly without the immune system as our guardian. But ongoing inflammation is what's really dangerous to your longevity. The toxic substances associated with the body's inflammatory response (its purpose is to eliminate living threats by killing them) means that over time your health is degraded, seriously.

The life-saving, killing process is termed "inflammation" because of the redness of the skin when there is a local infection. Seemingly simple, inflammation is series of complex biochemical processes that control the immune system's army of cells. The inflammatory substances dilate blood vessels in the skin to increase local blood flow—thus the red color—and attract white blood cells to migrate into the area. White blood cells consume the offending organisms and destroy them with their toxic substances.

The magnitude of the inflammatory response depends on the perceived magnitude of the threat. It can be local as with an abrasion or generalized. With a generalized acute infection, the response is systemic with fever and widespread aches and pains. Inflammatory substances are concentrated locally in localized infections but spread to the rest of the body as well in small amounts. In systemic infections, such as the flu, toxic substances are released in concentrations to make one sick.

These cytokines (cell-movers) are clinically significant inflammatory markers that are measured in the blood. The most common marker used in clinical medicine to indicate chronic infections is C-reactive protein (CRP). CRP is not just a marker of inflammation; it activates part of the immune system response to dead or dying cells. An easy way to remember CRP is that adding an A spells CR-A-P, which CRP is definitely not.

Everyone appreciates that increased bad cholesterol (LDL) is associated with increased vascular problems compared to those with lower LDL but even with an extended period of observation of those with high LDL only about half suffer bad vascular events. Markers of chronic inflammation are double in those with symptomatic vascular disease and quadruple in those who have had a heart attack. The most famous and trusted long-term study of cardiovascular disease in the world—the Framingham Heart Study—found that elevated CRP accurately predicted future cardiovascular events.[11]

Why Is Inflammation Harmful?

Our bodies are composed of trillions of individual cells whose overall functionality determines our health. Think of our bodies as compared to society in general; when the majority of citizens are healthy and gainfully employed everything is fine. In contrast, when an epidemic or recession incapacitates a significant percentage of the population, the society is impaired. Likewise with our cells; it depends to a large extent on the problem cell's function. Relatively small numbers of damaged cells in heart arteries can cause substantial harm, whereas non-cardiac muscle cells which are damaged may only be sore for a few days.

Aged cells gradually become less functional because over time the mechanism for sustaining life takes a toll. As mentioned in the earlier section on metabolism, the production of energy is a controlled chemical fire, producing sparks that are termed "free radicals." These offshoots damage vital parts of our cells, with damage occurring especially in the cellular furnaces (mitochondria) where the energy production takes place. The damage is as certain as death and taxes, but the rate at which the damage occurs is controllable. Readers of this book should recognize this and have a goal of reducing the rate of cellular damage.

Inflammation protects us and heals our wounds but it does this by increasing free radicals, which increases the pace of aging. Free radicals are caustic elements that are harmful to life—invading organisms and our cells as well. Inflammation increases local metabolism that is observable by intensified heat and, if sufficient, a fever develops. You could say, there is "collateral damage" from inflammation. The damage from short inflammatory states is minuscule but long-lasting inflammatory damage is cumulative and significant.

The sustained long-term inflammatory response's damage explains a great deal of the otherwise seemingly fragmented associations between lifestyle choices, aging, and protracted or chronic disease.

What Does Inflammation Have to Do with Aging and Lifestyle-Related Diseases?

Aging is not just the external signs we can see in the mirror: wrinkles, sagging chins, jowls, gray hair, or baldness. Those signs are the outward physical manifestations of our cells aging. The actual cellular aging process is complex and while we don't yet know everything about it we do know that chronic inflammation indicates the rate at which the ravages of aging worsen.

Recently researchers developed a method of calculating the age of a person's cells based on the length of the ends of their cellular DNA (telomeres). Using this method, the cellular age correlates with the level of inflammation quite well. More interesting, there is a rare genetic disease, Werner's disease, where adolescents begin to age rapidly and their cells are old when they are in their early twenties! People with this accelerated aging defect have significantly elevated markers of inflammation.[12]

Lowering inflammation reduces the rate at which we age and, conversely, we age faster when inflammation is increased. Smoking's low-grade inflammation worsens facial aging. Plastic surgery professors studied identical twins where one member smoked cigarettes and the other did not. Independent judges rated the wrinkles and looseness of skin in photos of the two groups and smokers were judged significantly older.[13]

More important than cosmetic aging, though, is the decline in function that can come with age. When sufficiently pronounced, the decline becomes the frailty syndrome.[14] There are five criteria for the syndrome: weakness, slowness, exhaustion, unintended weight loss, and low level of physical activity. The existence of any three of those criteria makes the diagnosis. The criteria for diagnosing frailty syndrome are important; four are symptoms of advanced aging and the fifth is likely a behavioral choice. I say likely because it could be that low level of physical activity was causal before it became mandatory.

Chronic inflammation is considered to be directly and indirectly, through obesity, related to the frailty syndrome.[15] Frailty predicts a systemic inadequacy of physiologic mechanisms; it is the herald of chronic disease's illnesses and the approach of the reaper. It is something you want to avoid.

You can see how chronic inflammation increases aging and its ravages and decreases longevity. The German Augsburg Cohort Study followed thousands of middle-aged men for 14 years and found those with elevated inflammation scores had double the overall death rates.[16] A study at the University of California likewise showed women with increased markers (CRP) of inflammation (>3) had eight times the vascular mortality of those with low levels (<1). CRP is the most commonly used test for detecting low-grade smoldering inflammation. When elevated, CRP predicts an increased chance of lung cancer, stroke, vascular disease, and Alzheimer's disease.

What Makes Aging Worse?

Smoking is quite possibly the worst accelerator of the aging process. Smoking irritates the largest organs in the body—the lungs. Amazingly, the lungs contain 1,500 miles of airways and if all the air sacks were flattened, the result would more than cover the floor of a two-car garage. In the Italian "Seven Countries Study," where lifestyles were studied for 40 years, smoking was the most detrimental to healthy longevity.[17] Men who smoked, ate unhealthy diets, and were sedentary died over a decade sooner, mostly from cancer, stroke, and heart attacks. Not desirable.

For four decades, I provided surgical care for some of the most lethal human diseases. Among the 12,000 patients on whom I performed cardiovascular surgery, I cannot recall a single person who did not have a lifestyle-induced risk factor. One patient was a pilot who was chosen to be an astronaut but because he had developed angina he was disqualified. On evaluation, I discovered he had severe coronary artery disease, which required a coronary bypass operation. This was a person who ran ten miles a day and had a Schwarzenegger-like body but he smoked cigarettes and dined mostly on fast food. It cost him the prize of a lifetime.

Exercise is very good at delaying aging-associated diseases. The idea of exercise, however, is too off-putting for some, or even rationalized as unnecessary. I was good friends with a famous surgeon who contributed greatly to medicine but who led a very unhealthy lifestyle. He smoked, drank, and frequently kidded me about my habit of regular exercise. "If you eat right and exercise," he would say, "you won't live longer, it will just seem that way." Once, he pointed out with certain smugness that a marathon runner had died of a heart attack during a race. "No one on the sidelines of that race died of a heart attack that day." He died of cancer at a younger age than I am currently.

A planned exercise routine, while important, is desirable but not essential. Just find ways throughout the day to be active. Being sedentary is the hazard. Sedentarianism is defined as expending less than 10% of energy-consuming activity in one's daily life. You don't want what it brings to your life.

A Swiss study defined moderate- and high-intensity activities among active people as sports such as tennis or skiing, or even walking, climbing stairs, gardening, and (for men only) occupational activities. In a Stockholm, Sweden, study more than 4,200 men and women were followed for 12 and a half years and their non-exercise activity levels noted. Those who were less active had higher rates of heart attacks and overall mortality. It's clear from scores of studies that inactivity accelerates decline that aging brings about.

What Makes Aging Better?

Healthy aging is aging while maintaining quality of life. There are three main pillars that support healthy aging. They are all lifestyle-related, which means you have the power to use them. They are, in order of importance: exercise, diet, and socialization. Each of these activities decreases inflammatory markers. Maintaining positive activity levels is the number-one preserver of a healthy body. Period. In the Whitehall II cohort study, almost 4,300 subjects were evaluated over the course of a decade.[18] The CRP levels in those who exercised for at least 2.5 hours per week remained lower and stable, while those who were less active saw CRP levels increase. In a Shanghai study, Dr. Wang administered the Aging Male Symptom Questionnaire to Chinese men and found those living healthier active lifestyles scored better on physical and sexual functioning.[19]

Over the last several decades, I personally have benefited notably from exercise; I feel better, look better, and am healthier as determined by functionality and by blood laboratory tests. I have spoken with numerous regulars at the gyms and they feel the same. When leaving off exercise for a few days, we find our mood and sense of self-worth decline.

My grandmother was an inspiration; she was a nurse by profession and a person who cared deeply for others, on and off the job. I never heard her complain about people who had done her wrong. She aggravated my Mom (who lived a few blocks away) because she would walk to the grocery store, which was several miles away, even in the Oklahoma summer heat, when Mom could have easily driven her. She tended a fine backyard garden and sewed quilts that she sold. Mostly, she stayed very active. She lived to be 101 years of age, fully able to care for herself, and stayed mentally alert. She simply went to sleep one night and didn't wake up. She lived a good, long life and experienced a good, short death.

Some scientists question whether exercise in the very elderly might be harmful because of their body's declining ability to withstand oxidative stress. The answer is that older bodies accommodate well and may even benefit more from physical activity than younger ones do. You'll find out more about the specific benefits of physical activity and exercise in chapter 6.

Diet can significantly reduce inflammation. Diet quality is measurable by the total nutrients (magnesium, vitamins A, C, and E, plus others) consumed. When the diet quality of low-income urban dwellers was measured in African Americans and whites, the higher the quality scores, the lower the inflammation.[20] Magnesium deficiency in particular has a strong association with inflammation in the elderly and may contribute to poor sleep patterns.[21] The diet supplies the body's fuel and building materials. These materials are what the body has to work with and that influence the body's metabolism, good or bad. You'll find in-depth information about diet in chapter 7. You'll learn, for example, that moderate alcohol consumption reduces inflammation and the advance of chronic disease.

The benefits of a rich social life have been examined in numerous long-term peer-reviewed studies and the findings repeatedly show that regularly scheduled social activities have significant beneficial effects on health and longevity. Chapter 8 provides you with some surprising information on this topic and will help you figure out how to increase your interactions in a way that works for you.

Periodontal disease is common and progresses for years with minimal warning symptoms. It is associated with elevated levels of inflammatory markers and prevalence of chronic diseases.[22] Spending a few minutes a day to brush, floss, and do regular dental cleaning can eliminate one common source of chronic inflammation.

I have had many patients and friends ask, sometimes jokingly: Why isn't there a healthy pill? Well there is; it's called aspirin. National Health and

Nutrition Examination Study found taking aspirin, along with a number of other factors, reduced inflammation.[23] Other studies with over 27,000 subjects including massive amounts of data found that long-term aspirin use reduced all-cause mortality, especially heart disease deaths and cancer.[24] Unfortunately, in biology, there usually is a drawback; aspirin not only reduces inflammation, it damages platelets, which stresses the clotting mechanism.

Aspirin is an acid and, if concentrated, can be caught in the stomach folds and erode the stomach lining. Regular aspirin dissolves rapidly and is more prone to cause stomach bleeding, whereas enteric-coated aspirin resists stomach acid for hours and thus passes beyond the stomach before releasing aspirin. There have been hundreds of studies to evaluate whether or not taking aspirin protects against age-related diseases. There is still some controversy but aspirin is clearly helpful in preventing heart attacks and stroke in those likely to suffer from those diseases. Taking low-dose aspirin reduces lung cancer and cancers of the gastrointestinal tract, especially colon cancer. Esophageal and gastric cancers are lessened by long-term regular aspirin ingestion. The cancers that aspirin prevents are some of the worst cancers in terms of the suffering they can cause. Get on board.

As mentioned, GI bleeding in the elderly is of concern. Low-dose (81 mg) enteric-coated aspirin, the recommended form, has a GI bleeding rate of less than 1% a year and most of these episodes are not fatal.[25] The Agency for Healthcare Research and Quality examined the risk/benefit ratio of regular aspirin consumption and concluded aspirin is beneficial in the elderly.[26] Those who have had GI problems and who are taking medications for chronic pain or blood thinners should not take aspirin without consulting their doctor.

Put Out the Fire!

You know it wouldn't be smart to leave a fall-cleanup brush-fire smoldering in your back yard; it could get out of control and burn down your house. Think of what you've learned about your body's immune system's chronic inflammation response in the same way—you don't want to burn down your body! So, take control. Take steps to make lifestyle choices that will improve your quality of life, increase your longevity, and help reduce your risk of developing chronic disease. Understanding the connection between chronic inflammation and aging is the first step toward a better and more successful way to maximize health.

Chapter 6

Clogged Pipes and Tire Blowouts

The Lifeblood of Vascular Disease

THE MAGNITUDE OF THE VASCULAR PROBLEM

Vascular disease will seriously impair the health or result in the death of one out of every two Medicare-age Americans. This means that vascular disease in one form or the other causes as much or more damage to the health of seniors than all other health problems combined. Isn't it sensible to know more about this pestilence of seniors?

Our cells depend on a steady uninterrupted supply of oxygen. In a matter of seconds of interrupted circulation, we will pass out and our hearts will sputter and stop. Without adequate oxygen-carrying blood flow humans don't survive very long.

"Vascular disease" is a broad term for a disease category that accounts for heart attacks, strokes, aneurysms, and gangrene. Vascular disease is universal after middle age; whether or not it initiates a major health crisis depends on how advanced it becomes. Many of the serious endpoints of vascular disease are lightning fast without warning. A person is well one minute and disabled or dead the next. Therefore, prevention is the key.

The skin is considered to reveal one's biological aging, especially the face. Generally speaking, facial aging is primarily from sun exposure and may not indicate vascular status. Vascular aging is much more dangerous and is from other lifestyle factors other than sun exposure. One's biological age is more important than one's chronological age. And, always remember your lifestyle impacts both, positively or negatively.

There is microscopic evidence of the beginnings of vascular disease in adolescence—called fatty streaking. During the Korean War, examinations of young soldiers' arteries that died in action showed a surprising amount of vascular disease. Gradually, this information provoked the realizations that high-cholesterol diets were not healthy as our mothers believed and smoking was not good for you as the actors posing as doctors in ads proclaimed. In people over 65, vascular disease is the most common cause of disability and death. Vascular disease should be taken very seriously.

Vascular disease has several presentations depending on the pathological process and the bodily region involved. As the title indicates, the pipes making up our circulatory system can clog up by plaque, clots, or both or develop weak spots leading to blowouts. Both are age and lifestyle dependent.

Our bodies are very dependent on a constant supply of oxygen and that means blood flow needs to be continuous; stopping the heart for as little as a few seconds will cause fainting. Our blood vessels are the living highways of pipes that carry oxygen to our cells. The greatest cause of death in America is vascular disease that reduces flow to body parts. In particular, as most know, heart attacks are the most lethal form of vascular disease.

VASCULAR DISEASE IS PERVASIVE

A key concept is that most everybody middle age or older has vascular disease in some stage of development, very similar to buildups in the pipes that make up your household plumbing. This vascular disease capable of causing blockages changes the way arteries feel to the touch; it changes them from soft and pliable to rock hard—thus, it is called arteriosclerosis (arterio = arteries, sclerosis = hardening). Ergo, its name means hardening of the arteries. There has been a naming of things in medicine using Greek and Latin names to aggrandize medicine which almost made me flunk first-year medical school.

These obstructions to free flow usually result from buildup of material, which is from repeated injury to the lining of arteries. Arteriosclerotic wounds can be produced experimentally in laboratory animals by damaging the arterial lining and giving drugs to raise their cholesterol. As the plaque slowly accumulates, it reaches a threshold where it causes blood flow to decrease. The point when flow becomes restricted is when the luminal diameter is reduced by half as seen on angiogram. This reduces the cross-sectional area by 70% when concentric. Since angiograms show the inside of arteries they are perfect for measuring inside diameters.

Blood flows can vary five or more fold from resting to vigorous exertion. Reductions in flow in heart arteries as flows need to increase can produce chest discomfort—called angina. More precisely, angina pectoris means literally angina—strangling—of the chest. The sensation produced is as if a weight is on the chest.

Angina is brought on by exertion or strong emotion, especially anger making the heart work harder, which requires more oxygen, thus requiring more blood flow. Imagine a lane or two of a multiple lane highway being closed. The obstruction to traffic flow would be far different during rush hour than in the middle of the night. Heart pain occurring at rest indicates far advanced disease.

Classic angina is in the middle of the left side of the front of the chest and may go down the left arm. Pain from our organs and pain from our skin are expressed by two different sets of nerves (somatic-skin and autonomic-organs) and they behave quite differently. As we all know, from needle sticks: the pain is sharp, identifiable as a needle stick, and is localized exactly to where it happened.

The autonomic (meaning without conscious control) nervous system perhaps should be called automatic because it acts automatically. And thank goodness because the thousands of functions our bodies do to provide us with breathing, heartbeat, digestion, sweating, and even sexual arousal don't require us to think about them; they are automatic—actually autonomic.

The downside is that the pain from organs may be vague, such as feeling like pressure when there is nothing pressing on the skin. The pain from the heart, located in the chest, may be felt in the upper abdomen or the jaw. One patient whom I put bypasses in his heart spent thousands on dental work before a correct diagnosis brought him to me. It is not uncommon for people having their first heart attack to think they have severe indigestion and thus delay treatment. And one-third of people have no heart pain at all, called silent ischemia which is dangerous because they have no heart warning system.

I have such a defective warning system. Because I knew from the Framingham Heart Study that one-third of men who dropped dead or had massive heart attacks had no warning, I started at 45 years to have heart stress tests every five years. I exercised daily since my youth, so I was greatly surprised when the stress test a decade ago was positive. But, hey, aging has its drawbacks. The next step when a stress test shows possible blockage is to get pictures of the inside of the heart's arteries (angiogram).

A cardiologist whom I knew performed the procedure, injecting dye into my heart's arteries. "Looks like God bypassed your arteries," he remarked when done. There is considered clinically to be three main arteries providing the heart with blood. I had one completely blocked and another closed off more than half. I should have had a massive heart attack and likely died.

The "God bypassed" statement was true, but nature bypassed or your healthy lifestyle would have been more accurate. The closed-off artery had newly formed a connection from an open artery (collateral vessel), which was as sufficient as a bypass. The 60% closed-off artery, the most important of the three heart arteries, was double normal size thus its flow was still adequate. My habit of continuing exercise from my youth had saved my life, just as scientific studies show will happen.

When not only pain from inadequate heart nutrition happens, but heart muscle dies, it is a heart attack. As everyone should know in this informa-tionage heart attacks kill more Americans than any other cause. Heart attacks occur when a diseased segment of artery abruptly closes because of a clot (coronary thrombosis). This is why low-dose aspirin has been shown to reduce heart attacks. Aspirin damages platelets in the bloodstream. Platelets initiate the clotting on damaged vascular walls. So, reducing the body's abil-ity to clot reduces clotting of diseased arteries.

The arteries have three distinct layers: an outer layer (the adventitia), a middle layer (the media), and an inner lining (the intima). The inside layer is important to our consideration of vascular disease. It is the Teflon of the vascular system. It is composed of the only cells (endothelium) that do not prompt blood to clot. As hardening of the arteries progresses, these important cells are damaged and do not cover the entire vascular surface. This exposure of uncovered vessel wall is a danger for clot to form, which can result in a heart attack. If you have not had a heart attack, behavioral changes can ward off this dreaded event.

Onset of chest tightness, difficulty breathing, jaw pain, or severe indigestion brought on by exertion or strong emotion should lead to medical evaluation of possible heart disease. The evaluation routine is standard. An electrocardio-gram that is unlikely to show anything is taken when the heart is not stressed and the heart pain is gone. Then because blood flow needs to increase oxygen availability with exertion a stress test is done. The most sensitive stress test is one injecting a radioisotope and scanning the heart after exertion. If the stress test is abnormal an angiogram is the gold standard because the pattern of disease is important in determining treatment.

It is widely assumed that when one has a heart attack one will know they are having a heart attack; this is often a false assumption. First, as shown by the most prestigious heart disease study, the Framingham Study, about one-third of men having their first heart attack have not had symptoms of heart disease because their nerves are hooked up so they do not have classical heart symptoms. They may experience no discomfort or have aching is uncharacteristic places, such as the stomach or jaw.

Heart and brain cells deprived of oxygen-containing blood die rapidly and the damage can be stopped by restoring blood flow. Not knowing when you have a serious problem that delays getting to medical care substantially increases risk of dying. The sooner a heart attack is treated, the less damage accrues. The average delay in arriving at an emergency room is over two hours. This is because the event may be considered indigestion, a toothache, or other non-serious problems. Often people having waited several hours because they think they have a stomach ache may die. The most common room for people to die in from a heart attack is the bathroom. In other not so essential areas such as the leg arteries failing, time also determines whether amputations are preventable or not.

HOW TO RECOGNIZE A HEART ATTACK

The symptoms of a heart attack come on suddenly. People often can time the attack to the minute. If something is very unexpectedly abrupt, it points to vascular causes. Sudden cold sweats, nausea and vomiting, profound weakness, extra heartbeats, and pain in the upper body for over five minutes should sound the alarm that something major is happening. Always, if in doubt, call 911. Paramedics can make the diagnosis and start treatment as they transport you to the hospital.

A neighbor called a while back complaining he did not feel well. He had given a pint of blood earlier in the day and was in his garden when he felt exceptionally weak in hottest summertime. He thought he was dehydrated which was logical. When I arrived he appeared exhausted, was sweating profusely, and was vomiting repeatedly. He also had extra heartbeats (premature contractions). He clearly was having an unrecognized heart attack. At the hospital he was taken immediately to the cath lab and treated. It was not a minute too soon; he was having serious heart rhythm problems that resolved when his main artery was opened.

Different patterns of blockages have different risks for serious heart damage from a heart attack. Treatment consists of two proven methods to restore blood flow: putting a catheter in the area of obstruction and inflating it. The procedure is an angioplasty (angio = artery, plasty = remodeling) or coronary artery bypass surgery where unessential blood vessels, arteries, or veins are used to go around the blockages. The bypass operations were used first and have been mostly superseded by angioplasty. Angioplasty squashes the plaque, reopening the heart vessel lumen. Expandable wire sheaths called stents are placed to keep the newly formed channel open. The first bypass surgery on heart arteries was performed at the Baylor College of Medicine in 1964.

THE ORIGIN OF HEART DISEASE TREATMENT

These treatments originated serendipitously at the Cleveland Clinic in 1958. Cardiac catheterizations were being done for valve and congenital heart disease but docs believed that to inject dye directly into the coronary arteries was dangerous and malpractice. Dr. Mason Sones was doing a study on a valve-diseased patient and the catheter slipped into a coronary artery and dye was injected. A perfect picture was obtained and the patient did well. Thus, Dr. Sones discovered coronary angiography that has helped many millions because once the coronary anatomy could be determined Dr. DeBakey's bypass surgery could be used to provide blood flow by going around the blockage. Yes, the disease is not removed. Instead, a new vessel is placed to provide flow around the blocked segment.

STROKES

Strokes result from the same mechanisms as heart attacks; the disease is in arteries in the neck not the heart. Strokes are not as deadly as heart attacks, but result in more disability than any other vascular disease.

What accumulates is called plaque; originally meaning "to stick," originally referring to an ornament you hung on the wall by sticking it there, then to material accumulating (sticking) on teeth or arteries. The plaque causing strokes is located in the arteries in the neck interfering with blood flowing to the brain.

The disease leading to a stroke may have warning symptoms. These are brief alarming symptoms of slurred speech, weakness of an arm or hand, or drooping of one side of the face. A take-home message is that symptoms from vascular insufficiency come on rapidly. One second you are normal and the next second not. These brain occurrences are from small clots breaking off from the plaque surface. They stick in small arteries temporarily interrupting blood flow and are known in medicine as transient ischemic attacks (TIAs). Should this occur medical help should be promptly sought to avoid a permanent loss of function.

Obstructions of the arteries located in the neck (carotid), causing strokes, are treated differently than heart disease. They are several times larger in diameter than the heart arteries and rather than obstructing from a clot as a primary cause of damage, they dislodge bits of clot. To remove this danger, the diseased carotid artery is opened (after being clamped off) and the inside layer carefully removed. A more recent therapy is to angioplasty and stent the diseased segment similar to treatment of heart arteries.

Hardening of the arteries may occur anywhere in the body and the manifestations of insufficient blood flow depends on the body part affected. The arteries to the legs are commonly involved (called peripheral vascular disease or PVD). The symptoms are comparable to those of heart disease. During brisk walking, the effected calf will cramp (intermittent claudication). Below the knee the leg arteries are small as the heart arteries and behave the same way. They are obstructed for a long period and then develop a clot that may completely close off and produce gangrene.

Before gangrene and beyond leg cramps, severe blockages can cause ulcerations, which don't heal. This is especially common in diabetics. Your doctor should be feeling your ankle pulses on your yearly physical examination and anytime you have leg cramps.

Tubes filled with fluid can not only become obstructed, they can weaken from pressure and dilates—similar to a weak spot with a bulge on a tire. The problem is evolution only protects our longevity until we procreate the next generation, then our survival is moot. Having diseased arteries occurs too late to influence evolution's genes. When arteries dilate, they become thinner and under relentless pounding of pulsatile flow, tend to rupture. Since loss of substantial blood volume is fatal, aneurysms are dangerous. Repair before rupture is not very dangerous but once ruptured aneurysms are quite lethal.

Aneurysms usually do not produce symptoms but if very large in the aorta they can cause back pain because they may erode the vertebral column. Any artery in the body can weaken and become an aneurysm. However, the most common sites are the aorta below the kidneys and inside the skull. Another cause of aneurysms is when the aorta develops a tear and blood separates the layers of its wall.

Dr. DeBakey and faculty members at the Baylor College of medicine developed the treatment for aneurysms and large vessel obstructions by replacing the diseased segments with cloth grafts. Dr. DeBakey was a leader in surgery at the beginning of aneurysm repair but the original repairs used aortas harvested from cadavers and were difficult to obtain, especially in the correct size.

Dr. DeBakey was a creative genius. He went to a department store, purchased a roll of a new cloth material, Dacron, that had just arrived, and used his wife's sewing machine to make tubes. The next day, he used a Dacron tube to repair an aneurysm and started modern vascular surgery. Dacron, as it turned out, was the best material for large vessel repair and is still used today—over half a century later.

Treatments for vascular disease as for most chronic diseases are technically well developed but they are expensive and their success rates depend on how far the disease has advanced and how much damage has accrued before treatment is started. A heart attack victim who has lost 40% of his or her left ventricular muscle will die. A stroke victim has lost neurons whose absence is responsible for whatever disability ensued. Those heart cells and neurons are gone forever. Any recovery, from rehab, is from other "recruited" neurons, which take over the function of those lost. This happens to varying degrees. Gangrenous limbs are gone permanently.

With the uncertainty that vascular disease presents with the risks to health and life, disruption of way of life, and often punishing costs, it is wise to employ preventive measures. Lifestyle measures are effective in preventing death from vascular disease.

The European HALE study observed almost a thousand men for a decade and observed death from heart disease according to lifestyle. The four-lifestyle criteria considered were: smoking or not, Mediterranean diet adherence, moderate alcohol, and physical activity.[1] Subjects having none or one of the good lifestyle criteria were lumped together. Those having two favorable behaviors were 40% less likely to have a heart attack; those with three 57% less likely; and those with all four were an incredible 73% less likely to have a heart attack. By easily attainable, lifestyle changes one can almost eliminate heart attacks. In the same study, all vascular deaths, mainly strokes after heart attacks, were reduced by 67%. A Greek study focused on over a thousand patients being treated for heart disease and found that those who adhered very slightly more to the Mediterranean diet survived significantly longer in a short period than those who ate unhealthily.[2] Even after a heart attack, introduction of an exercise program increased the chance of being alive in five years.[3]

There is no doubt that minimally disruptive lifestyle changes can improve survival by reducing danger from vascular disease—possibly even reversing it.

Chapter 7

Making Dementia Make Sense

Shoring Up the Senior Brain

Among all the aspects of aging that catch one's attention, developing dementia is the scariest. Gradually losing your selfhood which carried you through life and is the real "you" is unthinkable; not to mention discarding independent living. My Mom was a brilliant woman whose flashes of insight and encouragement propelled her three children living to adulthood into academic careers after they earned ten advanced degrees.

She was diagnosed as having Alzheimer's disease at the age of 81 years. I thank God that Mom never failed to recognize me. However, I am certain that she would not have wanted to live the last years of her life in the state she did. Now, we can plan ahead by knowing how to prevent or recognize early and deal with the dreaded dementia state.

THE INCREDIBLE BRAIN

The human brain is composed of the most amazing stuff and is the most complex material in the universe. It is three pounds of near jello consistency that is comprised of 100 billion nerve cells (neurons). These cells have long extensions that go from the brain to as far as the internal organs. They also have shorter extensions that are the business ends (dendrites, treelike in Greek). Our thoughts originate where two dendrites connect; they are living computer chips. The brain, through these connections, essentially functions like a binary computer but is much more. The truly amazing fact is that each of the 100 billion nerve cells can have as many as 10,000 connections. As we learn something new, more connections form. This equates to more neuron connections in a single brain than the number of minutes the Earth has existed. Big computing numbers give big computing capacity, which allows the human mind to do incredible tasks.

The human brain weighs more than other species except for elephants and whales. Further the design of the human brain is remarkable; it has hills and valleys producing twisted ridges on its surface called convolutions. The brainy ridges become more pronounced in higher primates and are associated in humans with greater intelligence.[1] This seemingly unlikely association has a good anatomical basis; brain cells form the gray matter of the brain and are located on the brain's surface. Convolutions increase the surface area of the brain, ergo, the more surface area, the more brain cells.

In the past, it was considered that unlike most other areas of the body, adults only lost nerve cells as we aged (rather depressing). However, the good news is that our grown-up brains have cells that die but our body forms new nerve cells as well.[2] Obviously we want to replenish more and lose less.

The aging brain decreases in size, especially in the frontal lobe areas and the hippocampus at the base of the brain. The hippocampus (hippo) decreases about 1% yearly after age 60 years.[3] This normal aging of the brain is very important because the function of the hippocampus allows one to lead an independent life. Actually, there are two of these small structures located at the base of the brain's right and left sides.

They are small, each averaging only the weight of a nickel (5 grams) but very important to overall functioning. The hippos retain very recent memory such as: Did I take my meds a few minutes ago? Did I turn off the stove? Where did I put my glasses? In other words, it allows us to live independently, thank goodness. Recent memory can be correlated with hippo volume.[4] Another necessary function the hippo has is spatial reasoning. When one goes into familiar places, the hippo recognizes and lets one know where they are located. It is a living Garmin GPS. When going somewhere it guides one back home. Also, the relationship between hippo size and dementia may or may not be causal but people with major depressive disorders have smaller hippos.[5]

The brain ages just like the rest of the body and the process changes mental functionality. None are exempt; we are all on the same conveyer belt. Normal brain aging usually allows independent living until the extremes of age. Thought processes gradually are slower, tending to be noticed when rapid decision making is necessary. Memory tends to be blunted especially in finding the right word or naming objects. It is normal aging if the forget-fulness is temporary. It is the "it'll come to me after a little while" episodes which signal normal aging. What the heck.

The balance center is located in the back of the brain at its base. Balance is less secure in the aging brain leading to a greater numbers of falls. Falls occur yearly in one of every three people over 65 years and one in three who falls will have serious injuries.[6] Not good odds. Recently, a vaunted, well-respected gentleman's life was ended at 96 years because of complications from a fall. He was an inspiration to all who knew him. He unfortunately spent the last few months of his life in rehab centers. His 93-year-old bride continues on bravely. They celebrated their 72nd anniversary two days before the fall.

Falls are the most common cause of death from injuries in the elderly. In 2013, according to CDC, over 25,000 deaths from falls were recorded. Falls generally are preventable with balance and strength training. Tai Chi is especially good to restore balance.

DISORDERS OF BRAIN FUNCTIONING

When the decline in mental functioning exceeds what should be considered normal for the person's age and educational level, a diagnosis of "Mild Cognitive Impairment" can be made. This impairment is present in 15% of people over 70 years of age.[7] It is not yet considered dementia because the disability is more of a nuisance that is not severe enough to interfere with daily living activities. It is considered a precursor for dementia, especially Alzheimer's dementia with 10–15% progressing to dementia yearly.

Mayo Clinic's outline of symptoms of individuals with Mild Cognitive Impairment is:

- You forget things more often.
- You forget important events such as appointments or social engagements.
- You lose your train of thought or the thread of conversations, books, or movies.
- You feel increasingly overwhelmed by making decisions, planning steps to accomplish a task, or interpreting instructions.
- You start to have trouble finding your way around familiar environments.
- You become more impulsive or show increasingly poor judgment.
- Your family and friends notice any of these changes.

Should one experience such indications, a medical evaluation is indicated. Should one suspect the development of mental disease, finding a physician knowledgeable on the subject to make an accurate appraisal is important. Family physician's awareness of patent's cognitive impairment was often wrong.[8] Your physician's office should be able to provide referral to the appropriate specialist. Use the knowledge of your primary care doctor's office to choose specialists. They refer to the best docs for certain conditions; they are a safety net, generally.

DEMENTIAS

The word "dementia" does not indicate a cause or define a particular disease; it indicates mental impairments, which are severe enough to disrupt normal living. In that regard, it is similar to the word "arthritis," meaning joint problems. Dementia derives from a Latin root meaning "out of one's mind." It is unsettling to even think about the suffering dementia causes.

There are six commonly recognized types of clinical dementia but Alzheimer's disease is overwhelmingly the most common (60+%, some estimates are as high as 80%) with vascular dementia a distant second at (15+%). The remainders of dementias are in low single digits; it is somewhat like the field of current republican candidates for president.

Dr. Alois Alzheimer was a German psychiatrist at the Frankfort Asylum who at 37 years of age in 1901 noticed a patient with unusual symptoms—Auguste Deter, a woman, 51 years of age. He became obsessed with her condition for five years until she died. He did an autopsy and made microscopic studies. Fortunately, the Germans were the most advanced in medical microscopy at that time.

The results were published in an obscure German medical journal. Other German psychiatrists confirmed Alzheimer's findings in their patients and when a popular medical book published the new disease, the new condition was named Alzheimer's disease and his fame was established. In medical history, I do not know of another case of fame so easily acquired.

Alzheimer's disease is particularly bad. Its cause is unknown; thus, it is incurable, it is relentlessly progressive, and ultimately destroys one's selfhood. It starts by interrupting pathways from the deposit of an abnormal protein in the brain's substance.

An index predicting the risk to develop Alzheimer's in people over their mid-70s is particularly accurate.[9] It includes factors indicating vascular disease such as those with evidence of carotid or coronary disease and those who do not drink alcohol. The study ran for six years. Four percent of the low-risk group developed Alzheimer's disease, while over 50% of those judged to be at highest risk came down with the disease.

Mild cognitive impairment (MCI) is often considered a precursor, as mentioned, to development of Alzheimer's. MCI patients who have small hippos have an increased risk of progressing faster to Alzheimer's.[10] It seems prudent to keep one's hippos as big and healthy as possible.

The American Psychiatric Association specifies three main criteria for the diagnosis of dementia: (1) memory impairment and impairment of at least one other cognitive domain (e.g., aphasia (speech problems), apraxia (motion problems), agnosia (sensory problems), or executive dysfunction (thinking problems)); (2) sufficient severity to lead to impairment in social or occupational function; and (3) decline from a previously higher level of functioning.

POSSIBLE WAYS TO PREVENT OR SLOW BRAIN AGING

Nobody wants to have dementia; it is a punishing, continually worsening nightmare. Dementia adds insult to injury because it has no cure in medical science. Dementia is alone in its devastation of not only the person affected but family and friends must suffer as well. Given the undesirability mentioned, prevention would be the only wise path to take. Denial is not an option. The statistics apply to all; none are exempt from the risk of dementia. Be aware and act proactively.

Scientific studies concerning prevention are of several types and each has differing reliability regarding health status or in this case mental status. First, there are observational studies, which examine the mental status as regards some aspect that may contribute in some way to the condition being examined.

As part of the aging process, the hippocampus shrinks by 1% a year after 65. This is why the annoying phenomenon of going into a room to retrieve something and forgetting why you are there becomes more frequent. The hippo is the first part of the brain to suffer in dementia. Because of spatial problems, an Alzheimer's patient may walk into a room and not only forget the why; they can forget where they are which is why they often wonder off or go for a walk and forget how to return—a most frightening feeling.

I lived in Houston for years and rarely went downtown. Then I had an occasion to go to an appointment in the center of downtown and set my GPS for the address. The skyscrapers blocked the functioning of the GPS and I was lost in the valleys between the skyscrapers and busy one-way streets. It was a most disagreeable feeling.

The most physically fit have the largest hippos. One study took a group of elderly subjects and started some on exercise programs. They measured both group's hippos after a year and found the exercise group's hippos did not decrease as did the control group; their hippos unexpectedly increased in size.[4] On average, two years of hippo shrinkage was reversed!

Vitamins and supplements have mixed results in studies and possibly because of the money involved, pharmaceuticals are far more often studied. However, a well-done multiethnic study determined vitamin D status in normal and demented subjects who were followed for up to 8 years.[11] Subjects with low vitamin D levels had both normal and diseased brains which worsened more over time than subjects with adequate vitamin D. The authors made the disclaimer that the data did not determine that vitamin D supplements would be protective. However, taking proper doses of vitamin D has no downside and quite possibly would slow mental decline.

Statins have been shown to reduce the chance of getting Alzheimer's disease by about half in the elderly.[12] This is in comparison to people with elevated cholesterol without statin therapy. But statin therapy also is protective in people with normal cholesterol who do not need statins. Correlation does not prove causation. For instance an observational study could be designed to correlate the possibility of violence from carrying a gun with the color of one's clothes would certainly show blue to be correlated because police mostly wear blue. This may change with the growth of concealed carry.

Healthy lifestyles have repeatedly been shown to promote brain health and preserve mentation. The questionability of this data is that the studies are often observational, that is a group of subject's lifestyles are correlated to their mental status and whether or not they have dementia. The fault is that people who exercise may do so because they have better preserved brains or they may indeed be more health savvy.

Social isolation is bad for one's brain. Living alone versus being married and living with someone almost doubled the chance of becoming demented.[13] This well-done study was completed on elderly adults in Sweden and published in a premier medical journal. Conversely, the National Long-Term Care Survey examined the cognitive decline of older people over a 10-year period according to their exercise routines, cognitive activities, and socialization.[14] They unfortunately found only exercise to be significantly better in preventing mental decline. However, the end points were different and the subjects were somewhat younger.

Physical activity has always been considered the best insurance policy against developing Alzheimer's disease. Extensive medical literature shows significant protective effects.[15] Over 2,000 elderly (71–90 years) men were studied in Hawaii as to their risk for developing Alzheimer's and their average daily walking distance.[16] Those who walked least, less than a quarter of a mile daily, were 80% more likely than those who walked more than 2 miles daily to develop dementia. Two miles total over a day is not a lot.

A study in Spain randomized elderly subjects into a Mediterranean diet group supplemented with olive oil or nuts and a control group.[17] They had repeat cognitive testing after six years and the healthier diet group had less cognitive decline. An observational study ranked normal older people according to diet, finding that those who ate more healthy fats and green vegetables had a 38% less chance of developing Alzheimer's during the study period.[18]

In a French study, naturally French, moderate consumption of alcohol decreased dementia by 42%.[19] Interestingly, *the form of the alcohol intake had no influence in prevention.* These data run counter to the popular belief that red wine is the only protective form of alcohol because of the resveratrol red wine contains.

In a Finnish study the scientists enrolled over 2,000 subjects and randomized them into a group that were exposed to multiple healthy lifestyles including diet, exercise, cognitive training, and vascular risk modification. The comparison group continued their regular routines. After only a two-year period, the change in mental abilities was significantly better in the intervention group in normal, mild cognitive impairment, and dementia.[20] Multiple lifestyle interventions stopped the mental decline of aging. And this study was published in one of the most prestigious and selective journals on the planet.

A New York City study examined the effect of both exercise and diet on the risk of getting Alzheimer's dementia in a 12-year observation period.[21] They found, as one might hope, the benefits were additive, as is shown repeatedly in many studies. Each healthy lifestyle's contribution added to reducing the chance of Alzheimer's tragedy from rearing its ugly head to mar one's golden years.

Part II

LIFESTYLE CHANGES AND PREVENTION

Chapter 8

Lifestyle-Related Ailments

Living Better Longer

WHAT EXACTLY IS LIFESTYLE?

Lifestyle has the simplest definition for one of the most complicated doings possible. Lifestyle is simply the particular way an individual or group choses the living style they wish to embrace. I realize the words "life" and "living" are considered synonyms. But in this overview, life and living differ. Living is a consolidation of experiences involving many choices, whereas life is the biochemical phenomenon which is unbelievably complex and which keeps us alive so we can live. How we choose our living to go, ergo lifestyle, profoundly influences our life-giving apparatuses. To a profound extent, these apparatuses determine how long and how well our living goes.

I previously used the metaphor of a swimming pool. The living process is the water in our swimming pool; our lives are filled by the important things. The solid material "pool" (our lifestyle) simply contains the essential thing. We ignore its importance because, as the water in our pool, it is just there. How we manage the water in our pool profoundly determines the quality of the pool.

Regarding health, the old saying "it's who you know, not what you know" is backward. Actually, concerning health it's what you act on about what you know that matters. Those of you reading this book are successful and success depends on acting on and following through on what you know, mixed with a portion of deferred gratification. I mix in deferred gratification because it is a necessary trait for success in any endeavor.

When one goes to exercise leisure activities are suspended. I feel better by exercising for a period of time than watching a meaningless TV show. I get more benefit by consuming a lean-high antioxidant meal than a high-fat diet with a high carb soda. My luck with grades came at about one o'clock in the morning studying a subject rather than snoozing. Apply the same grit to your health lifestyle. You will be rewarded more than you know.

Lifestyle improvement disappears when considered an all-or-nothing situation. Although worsening may be sudden and severe, improvement is incremental, which is why five out of six who started exercise programs failed to continue long term. Starting slow and gradually increasing is a good strategy.

Lifestyle means deciding healthy and taking actions that equate with those choices. Your health is too important to take the Iranian approach: doing whatever you want and declaring it OK.

TOO MUCH TAKING IT EASY IS BAD

"Sedentary" is a nine-letter dirty word. It applies to an individual when 10% or fewer calories are consumed from activity.[1] There is clearly indisputable evidence that sedentary individuals have decreased longevity by getting some of the deadliest diseases such as heart disease and cancer. Also, sedentary behaviors increase some of the most undesirable ones such as depression and dementia.[2]

A sedentary lifestyle can lead directly to the frailty syndrome, which has an awful prognosis.[3] The unwanted diagnosis requires any three of the five criteria: (1) generalized weakness, (2) slowness, especially walking, (3) low level of physical activity, (4) self-reported exhaustion, and (5) unintentional weight loss. The frailty syndrome is seen in 7% to 12% of people over 65 years; so, the syndrome is fairly common.[3] "Currently, exercise and comprehensive geriatric interdisciplinary assessment and treatment are key interventions for frailty."

Nurses' Health Study measured telomere (telo = ends, meres = things; ends of chromosomes that determine the age of the cells) length in over 7,000 nurses and the telomeres in active nurses were significantly younger than in the sedentary.[4] They concluded that "Although associations were modest, these findings suggest that even moderate amounts of activity may be associated with longer telomeres." This is a well-done study but is observational, meaning it is suggestive but inconclusive. What follows are several "controlled" studies that can be used to make reliable conclusions.

In a Spanish study, over 2,700 sedentary subjects over 60 years were encouraged to increase their activity levels.[5] Those following a moderate program had a one-third lower mortality over the next few years and those who were rigorous lowered theirs by almost half.

Sedentary behaviors are correctable by increased activity. A minimum threshold to get improved mentation is 45 minutes of exercise at least twice weekly.[6]

A European study of older, overweight sedentary people's telomeres had remarkable findings.[7] Half were started on an increased physical activity program and half remained sedentary. In only six months the exercisers' telomeres were significantly better. Wow.

SOCIAL ISOLATION: ONE IS THE LONELIEST NUMBER

Humans are social-focused creatures. Most of us don't like to spend excessive time alone unless we are engaged in a task, which occupies our attention. A well done study in the Kungsholmen district followed for three years older non-demented subjects living at home.[8] During the study about 10% developed dementia. The incidence of dementia was doubled in single people living alone without social networks. They concluded: "An extensive social network seems to protect against dementia." Residents in residential senior living quarters psychologically deteriorate over time. Forming ladies' and men's clubs reversed this and gave a sense of well-being.[9]

The following is taken from a 2012 article in U.S. News and World Report: "I think one of the major issues for adults as they get older is to maintain their social connection," says Colin Milner, CEO of the International Council on Active Aging (ICAA) in Vancouver. "An example of this is the fact that 70% of baby boomers see retirement as a time when they want to spend more time with their families. Yet people can often get isolated as friends and family move away or pass on. This can become a significant issue, leading to depression and a downward spiral with one's health." The social withdrawal combined with lack of concern about surroundings, occasionally with excessive accumulation of things, is the Diogenes Syndrome which results in a high mortality rate.[10]

Diogenes of Sinope is one of my favorite Greek philosophers. He was one of a kind; he lived alone in a tub, totally unconcerned about surroundings, and searched perpetually for an honest man—failing to find one.

As people age, retiring and becoming frail are possible turning points where social contacts and participation can wane. This must be avoided because those times are when support and self-awareness are the most important.

Improve Your Sleep and be Refreshed

Sleep is included not because it is normally classed as a lifestyle mode but because it is a lifestyle determinant. Sleep is another way of enhancing or depreciating life and therefore affects lifestyle. Suitable sleep is an important part of our lifestyles; it is the balm of our mental and physical being. It recuperates us from the daily wear and tear of living.

Sleep is a time of replenishment; it builds up our nervous, immune, bone, and muscular systems. It also, probably because of our recumbent posture, eliminates excess water. During sleep even when dreaming, the brain is idling; normally *the brain although only three pounds uses 20% of our energy.* Sleep allows the brain to replenish energy (Adenosine Tri-phosphate [ATP], our body's gasoline), which makes us awake refreshed and eager to meet a new day.

Insomnia is the prolonged and usually abnormal inability to get enough sleep. It includes being unable to fall asleep, stay asleep, or awakening too soon. As a result of these forms of insomnia, the quality of your sleep is poor, which makes you tired during the day and leads to a need for increased medical care.

Between 10% and 30% of people report sleep problems.[11] Obesity is associated with sleep apnea but not with sleep difficulties in general.[12]

There is a particularly bad form of sleep deprivation that may not be noticed by the sleeper—sleep apnea. According to the NIH, "Sleep apnea (AP-ne-ah) [without breath in Greek] is a common disorder in which you have one or more pauses in breathing or shallow breaths while you sleep. Breathing pauses can last from a few seconds to minutes. They may occur 30 times or more an hour. Typically, normal breathing then starts again, sometimes with a loud snort or choking sound. Sleep apnea usually is a chronic (ongoing) condition that disrupts your rest from sleep because of the repeated interruption of the oxygen supply. When your breathing pauses or becomes shallow, you'll often move out of deep sleep and into light sleep." It usually disrupts the sleep of someone nearby.

Sleep apnea is a leading cause of excessive daytime sleepiness. Recurrent insomnia is associated with poor quality of life and increased need for medical care. It is more than just an annoyance. The danger is that sleep apnea increases the risk of arrhythmias, myocardial ischemia/infarction, stroke, and heart failure, all of which may increase mortality risk.[13] Sleep apnea should definitely be evaluated by a sleep medicine doctor. Symptoms are obvious, sometimes disturbingly so, to a loved one close by. Sleep apnea requires professional help.

Although insomnia is common, most do not have serious problems. These are mostly intermittent in nature and possibly improved by the following counsel which is a composite from various sources including Harvard, Mayo Clinic, and the University of Maryland sleep centers and WebMD.

1. Have a regular routine for going to bed. Retire at the same time and go through the same preparations (possible examples are): set up coffee, take meds, dental hygiene, stretching, or reading.
2. Exercise routines help considerably. Avoid exercise late in the evening.
3. Increase exposure to sunlight during the day and evening.
4. Avoid long naps, particularly after 2:00 p.m. Limit naps to 1 nap of less than 30 minutes a day.
5. Maintain restful temperature in bedroom. Usually on the cooler side.
6. Decrease light and noise exposure as much as possible. Lower the shades or use blackout curtains.
7. Limit liquid intake for several hours before bedtime.
8. Be aware of effects on sleep of any new meds.
9. Relax and put off worry until tomorrow. Meditate or vent your feelings to a loved one if anxious.

The National Health Aging Trends Study examined sleep habits in more than seven thousand elderly and found social activities with a good network reduced insomnia by two-thirds, regular exercise by more than half, and both dropped insomnia by even more. So, become an exercising socializer or a socializing exerciser.

PRINCIPLES OF AN ANTIAGING DIET

Overall dietary principles include proper intake of protein and fiber and reduction of salt but this theme focuses on an antiaging diet. Lifestyle concerning diet is important but the proper dietary lifestyle can be summarized by three recommendations.

The first is calorie control. The average calorie content of restaurants, both chain and non-chain, are excessive being double the requirement for health.[14] It is rare my bride or I finish an entire meal alone when eating out. Instead, depending on circumstances, we split a meal or, by design, eat half and box the rest. We get a bargain-basement deal when eating out.

When at home use smaller plates and fill them with two-thirds of what you consider a portion. If you remain hungry, you can always eat more. Okinawans don't say grace before meals; they say "eat until you are 80% full." They are the longest-lived people on the planet. As you adjust volume of intake down, your body will be satisfied with less and you will feel full sooner.

Caloric restriction extends the healthy life of all living creatures thus tested by as much as 30% even in primates.[15] Rhesus monkeys on reduced calories versus animals who ate all they wanted looked years younger and were much more alert and active; their youth was preserved.

LOCATING THE BAD ACTOR FOODSTUFF

Among the three foodstuffs, carbohydrates (sugar), amino acids (protein), and fat, fat gets the bad rap and if habitually taken in excess, damage to your body occurs but damage is primarily from increasing the size of one's fat cells. *Sugars are the potentially harmful molecules.* We are alive because of a controlled chemical fire in our cells. It is a form of oxygenation (combining with an oxygen atom), which describes forest fires, gasoline engines, rust, and our cell's fires—termed "respiration" if occurring in our cells. Sugar unlike coal must be burned when received.

Blood sugar needs to be kept within narrow limits. Insulin regulates blood sugar by forcing it into cells. The more sugar consumed, the more insulin secreted and the more sugar forced into cells which must "burn" it. More intense hotter cellular fires release more sparks and at a certain rate the number of harmful molecules exceeds the body's protective mechanisms.

It is not just the amount of sugar containing food or drink consumed (sugar load); it is how fast the sugar is absorbed, termed the "glycemic index" (GI). The index is set at 100 for pure sugar. Low GI foods rate below 55 and above 70 is considered high.

There are two advantages to low GI foods: they reduce the amount of damage from excess sparks and they are more satisfying longer. High GI foods lead to a rapid peak sugar level that dips lower and causes the consumer to feel hungry and predisposes to overeating. The GI of almost 3,000 non-diabetic subjects was determined and they were followed for 4.7 years.[16] A high GI increased the mortality rate from all causes. From epidemiological studies there is incomplete evidence that artificial sweeteners increase cancer risk, especially aspartame.[17]

The antidote for sparks is molecules that serve as "fire extinguishers" called antioxidants. The sparks (oxidants) indiscriminately attach to other molecules inside the cell where they were formed, causing damage. Antioxidants attach selectively to oxidants neutralizing them. Then they are safely eliminated in the urine. Thus, the third principle is to eat foods high in antioxidants. These foods include beans, berries, most fruits (especially grapes) and vegetables (dark green and tomatoes), nuts from trees (walnuts, pecans), and sweet potatoes. ***Bon appetit.***

Chapter 9

The Magic of a Dynamic Life

How to Get Your MOJO Back

"MOJO" is a magic word. It originally meant a magic spell or amulet to achieve a desired end. Now MOJO recognizes that there is an underlying vibrant meaning to experiencing a lively right-on life. It shouts "I can do it" to no one in particular because it is internal, but knowing that, the external manifestations will be observed by others. The great Muddy Waters popularized MOJO in 1957 in the classic "Got my Mojo Working," which he pronounced "wurkin." If you have forgotten your MOJO, watch John Travolta dance in *Saturday Night Fever* and you will remember.

American Heritage Dictionary gives several definitions, one of which is: "An ability or quality that causes one to excel or have good luck." Those of us that are older consider the very best capability granting good luck is to maintain a quality of life that gives us pleasure and allows independence, but MOJO even goes beyond that; it beckons us to be proud of what we can do. This includes mental, physical, social, spiritual, and, yes, sexual roles, all of the arenas that make life worthwhile.

MOJO is not just something wonderful wasted on the young. The advantage of maintaining a good quality of life accrues more benefits as we age because we have less reserve to relinquish. Keeping MOJO is choosing to lead a dynamic, vigorous life. The key word is choosing.

Ageism is rampant and it is as negative as other -isms. Ageism implies that growing older means unavoidable deterioration and therefore decreasing worth. It is a false idea. The elderly are not able to function as if they were twenty but they do not need or desire to do so. They can function superior to then because of increased knowledge and wisdom allowing better judgment. However, whatever one's age, they want to function at a level that meets their needs: physically, mentally, spiritually, and socially. MOJO is the knowing you can do what you want to do. Maintaining functional MOJO guarantees well-being in these needs.

The average time in a professional football player's career is six seasons. George Frances Blanda, NFL Hall of Famer, played for 26 seasons. He was a great quarterback/place kicker and gave us this wisdom: "I never threw [the football] in the offseason. I've been around so long, I could be blindfolded and spun around a dozen times and still know where the goalposts are." That should become our objective, to know where the goalposts are located—definitely; always go for the gold. Blanda kept a steady physical, social, and mental routine; he never misbehaved, as a lot of professional athletes do. There is a lot to learn from those who maintained their MOJO: stay active in the spheres of function that are desirable and the functions will continue to be available. Science's crystal ball provides us ways to maintain our MOJO.

Back two and a half millennia, half a millennium before Jesus, Hippocrates, the father of medicine, noted, "Walking is man's best medicine"; ever since, all evidence, subjective, empirical, and rigidly scientific, strongly, without exception, has supported that contention. "Exercise" is not a dirty word; it is very positive. The *Merriam Webster Dictionary*'s definition of exercise is: "physical activity that is done in order to become stronger and healthier." So, exercise is activity with a worthy purpose.

Animals are made to be mobile, unlike plants whose job it is to be biological solar panels; animals need to forage for fuel. Until the arrival of agriculture and animal husbandry, our hominoid ancestors had to be physically active in acquiring food. Except for certain times of year and certain choice locations, those who caught more game ate more and had increased survival, likely because they traveled greater distances foraging. Now human's greatest foraging problem is standing in line at the checkout stand. Incidentally, never get behind me at checkout; I always pick the slowest most-problematic line.

The most successful human hunters obviously were those who could cover the greatest distances most quickly. Better hunter's survival advantage is to possess more active cellular furnaces producing more damaging free radicals as we understood from the chapter on metabolism. In biology, all energy production and hormonal systems that potentially can go out of control have mechanisms to limit excesses. Antioxidant generation limits excess free radicals. Our ancestors who were better hunters and survived developed better antioxidant generating bodies. This was passed on to us.

So, it seems paradoxical for exercise to benefit the body since it tremendously increases the cellular energy level and thus increases the harmful free radicals generated. Free radicals are the sparks from the chemical cellular fires we discussed earlier. Similar to actual sparks, they can damage surrounding structures. Free radicals measurably increase after exercise but the enhancement of the body's defense mechanism of producing neutralizing substances by regular workouts occurs.[1]

The *balance between the amount of harmful free radicals and mechanisms of neutralizing antioxidants is the important concept.* In nature, every damaging bodily process has a means of counteraction for survival. As an example, when we are in danger hormones are secreted to make our bodies stronger and faster but our bodies have counter measures to shut down the process when no longer needed because unchecked, stress hormones could kill us. There are rare tumors of the adrenal glands where stress hormones are manufactured which produce stress hormones in abundance. Unless removed those with these tumors will die very early. As will people who are under constant stress.

The counter measures for free radical sparks are enhanced by exertion, more than needed to neutralize the damage. Exercise activity deposits health certificates in your body's bank account.

The damaging state of oxidative stress occurs when there are more damaging substances than can be dealt with by the body. Concerns that the elderly might be damaged by exercise are disproven; the elderly benefit more than younger people from exercise.[2]

Evidence for the beneficial effects of exercise began thousands of years ago, as uncovered by anthropologists. There have been comparisons of fossils from hunter/gatherers and other ancients soon after the agricultural age began. Determining anything from prehistoric bone fragments is inexact but the more active hunter/gatherers fossils had signs of being healthier as compared with farmers, especially their teeth and long bones. Hunters lived longer and had healthier offspring. It is assumed that since the diets differed between the two groups, diet has some effect but hunter/gatherers were constantly walking, their lives depended on finding game. Chimpanzees are usually imagined lounging about as in zoos but in the wild, they average foraging almost 10 miles daily. Also, berries, nuts, and other foodstuffs were seasonal and often required hunter/gathers relocating, without cars. We know activity is good, otherwise why do people walk their dogs?

Everyone knows exercise is beneficial, yet studies show that only one-third of Americans declare that they exercise regularly.[3] And since the exercise duration in the quoted study was only ten minutes or more, probably half of those do not exercise with enough vigor or long enough to secure health benefits. Error in surveys that ask whether one does something desirable is usually skewed upward with people claiming desired behaviors they do not actually do.

Fortunately, I started to exercise regularly before jogging was popular. I started boxing when young and built stamina through roadwork. The endorphins enhanced my mood, so I continued to the present day. Because the Framingham Heart Study showed that one-third of men had their first heart attack without ever experiencing angina as a warning, even though I exercised daily, at 45 I had a heart stress test, which was negative. I went fourteen minutes and my friend the attending cardiologist complained, "I should have brought a book." When I had a repeat stress test about 15 years later, I was astounded to learn it was positive.

As protocol recommends, a catheterization was done which showed one artery closed and another with over 50% constricted, a situation usually requiring surgery but the partly blocked artery was twice normal size and the blocked artery had a huge new vessel supplying it. The cardiologist amazedly remarked, "It looks like God bypassed your heart." My body solved a serious chronic disease problem. An adult lifetime of healthful lifestyles paid off—otherwise, I should be dead.

The most obvious importance from exercise is that those who exercise live longer. A Harvard Alumni study showed that physical activity consuming over 1,500 calories a week, a total of about three to four hours of moderate exercise, reduced risk of dying more than stopping smoking.[4] This finding makes exercise the most powerful health-promoting behavior.

In another large study of 19,000 subjects over 65 years, total mortality was significantly reduced by exercise. Moreover, the degree of reduction depended on the intensity and duration of the exercise.[5] As the amount of moderate exercise increased, the chance of dying reduced proportionally.

Moderate exercise means that benefits require crossing a threshold. In the Nurses' Health Study, walking benefits began to be significant at three miles per hour. The study determined a threshold of three miles an hour by having subjects adjust the speed of a treadmill to the speed they normally walked. They then followed the large group of thousands for years and found mortality was reduced by almost half from heart attacks.

What is the danger of exertion causing a fatal heart rhythm? Sudden death from vigorous exertion can occur but is exceedingly rare; according to the Nurses' Health Study one death happened in 36.5 million hours of exertion.[6] This incredibly low statistic fell further if subjects were exercising regularly two or more hours a week.

The greatest health benefit from a regular exercise program, besides improved functionality, is on the arteries. At first, this seems paradoxical because during moderate to intense exercise, the blood pressure can elevate rigorously. However, in the fit individual, it rapidly returns to baseline and overall regular exercise tends to lower blood pressure when not exerting.

"A person is as old as their arteries are" is a truism. Arterial blood flow keeps one's community of cells alive and functioning. Failures because of obstructions cause heart attacks and strokes, the number one and number four causes of death in America, respectively; combined they are half of the top five causes of death, and they originate from largely preventable vascular disease.[7] Everyone has vascular disease which slowly worsens but by exercising one pushes back the age when the disabilities of major vascular events occur.

Stroke is the number one cause of disability in America. Low fitness is one of the strongest predictors of future stroke.[8] Nothing in biology is 100% but a regular exercise program, of sufficient intensity and frequency, is the best assurance of better health, better life, and a better death.

One caution about starting an exercise routine is that heart attacks are often triggered by episodic physical and sexual exertion in people who do not exercise regularly.[9]

So, it would be wise to check with a physician to determine safety and to start slow with incremental increases in exertion. All benefits are incremental and accrue over time. The incremental nature of health and disease is a foundational principle of this book. Incremental things must be evaluated over time. As your retirement nest egg grew monthly. But every ten years the amount was amazing. Health is glacial in change—one way or the other (glaciers average moving a meter a day).

Gyms across the country have influxes of new enrollees occasioned by "New Year's Resolutions." Serious exercisers bear the increases in exercisers at the beginning of the year but by spring, superficial resolutes are gone. Their expectations of rapid remodeling did not materialize. Almost all detriments or benefits to physical and mental health are incremental. Imperceptible changes occur exercise period by exercise period. An athlete spends years of training to reach an extraordinary level of performance, incrementally. One does not graduate from business school and get hired as the CEO; everything in life is incremental. And a cigarette smoker almost always must consume tobacco daily for over 20 years before lung cancer develops, incrementally. Changes in our bodies are gradual, just as a huge cathedral is built, brick-by-brick. Thus, although health markers increase in weeks from starting an exercise program, benefits accumulate slowly but invariably.

Living longer is a blessing only when the quality allows an enjoyable life worth living. Exercise has been shown to decrease the ravages of aging, which has been equated with capturing a longevity dividend.[10] Elderly citizens maintaining their own residences were followed for four years. Those who walked daily were less likely to develop dementia or other problems requiring nursing home placement. One study started community exercise programs in elderly persons and found them, a year later, to be more fit and functional than before.[11] Amen.

The Dijon Three Center Study is exceptionally convincing of a healthy lifestyle's benefits on quality of life in the elderly.[12] Almost 4,000 subjects with no disability were followed for 12 years, according to criteria of a healthy lifestyle and whether they became disabled or not. Four simple criteria are used: smoking; little physical activity; consuming less than one helping of fruit and vegetables daily; and heavy alcohol drinking. All except alcohol consumption were associated with increased disability. Smokers with a bad diet and little activity increased their disability two and a half times!

Mental functioning in over 18,000 nurses in subjects over the age of 70 years revealed that the more the elderly exercised, the better was their mental sharpness.[13] In addition, when the study continued, exercisers had less decline over a six-year observation period. Those benefiting walked at least 1.5 hours per week, which is a good return on one's time spent.

It is well known that regular exercise reduces a variety of mental pathology. Worth repeating, the part of the brain responsible for recent memory, the hippocampus, shrinks 1–2% yearly in the elderly. The loss of hippocampal volume is considered responsible for memory loss and in an advanced state for dementia. Using MRI measurements of brain structure, it has been verified that these vital brain structures are larger in people who maintained physical fitness.[14]

Scientists studied the hippocampal volumes of elderly subjects (over 65 years) Which were divided into two groups: one group was assigned to do an aerobic exercise routine three days a week and the other comparable group did stretching exercises. At the end of one year, the hippocampal measurements were repeated and compared individually and between the two groups. Individuals who stretched had the usual 1–2% decrease in hippocampal volume, whereas those utilizing aerobic exercise did not decrease; *surprising the investigators, their hippocampi increased in size and accordingly their cognition tests improved.*[15] Exercise made their hippos a year or two younger.

Mental health in general is improved by regular exercise. Adult subjects who exercised daily for four weeks and others who exercised only on test day showed improved cognition, decreased anxiety, and elevated mood with regular exercise.[16] The key word is "regular." The body needs time to adjust. The authors found that beneficial brain factor (neurotropic factor) which has a protective effect on brain aging was increased with regular exercise. Enhancement of mental functioning and mood was found with aerobic exercise; strength training did not show any benefit in mentation.[17]

Aerobic exercise went beyond reducing the chance of developing mental illness; regular exercise predicted that one would be more satisfied with life.[18] When scientists recorded a group of elderly subjects' activities and administered a Satisfaction with Life Scale, the extent of their activity correlated positively with quantifiable contentment. A large study in Spain looked at whether or not an appreciable amount of leisure time was spent in physical activity. Among other benefits, those with physical activity had better social functioning and emotional stability.[19]

One concept of aging, termed "ageism" is the negative perception toward the elderly by others, including the elderly themselves. Age, according to ageism, past the middle years, and also in adolescence, is considered to be lacking complete mental functionality.

This opinion of hypothetical elderly persons by others was significantly upgraded if the subjects were described as being physically active and was proportional to the activity level described.[20] In other words, when older people are viewed as being more functional, the ageism concept became less negative and the subjects were considered as younger and more positive, the more active they were described.

A sedentary lifestyle ensures a greater chance of masculine erectile dysfunction.[21] This is the dreaded ED. Even when the relationship between ED and exercise in younger healthy males is studied, erectile performance is improved in the more active men.[22] Also, sexual satisfaction was increased in those exercising. Enhancement of erectile function has been seen repeatedly in the elderly and obese who are active but the unhealthy would be more likely to have both decreased physical and sexual function. Could the association be phallus-acious? A note of caution is in order for over-the-counter supplements to relieve sexual dysfunction. Studies have found that many have adulterants which may be harmful.[23]

Scientists, in a well-done study, recruited a group of men with ED and instructed half on exercise and diet; the other half were given dietary instructions alone.[24] All subjects had discernible both erectile and sexual dysfunction (other performance issues) as determined by the International Index of Erectile Dysfunction. The "Index" has 15 intimate questions with a perfect score of 75 points. At the start, all the subjects had scores below 21, indicating definite dysfunction. After two years, one-third of those instructed in exercise had lessened markers of inflammation and considerably improved sexual function. Another study showed ED harbingered generalized vascular disease (heart attacks and stroke) and all three, including ED, could be overcome by initiating both exercise and a healthy diet (Mediterranean diet).[21]

A side issue is the association of ED and the decrease in a body substance that regulates blood flow (nitric oxide, NO for short). The body manufactures NO and it becomes reduced as we age. Erection takes place because blood flows into the important male love gland (penis, scientifically) and NO makes the increased flow possible. Viagra and other ED meds increase NO and, thus, allow erection to occur.[25] NO is produced from an amino acid, arginine, which can be purchased as a supplement. NO also is considered to increase hormones that build muscle and increases hormones that may be decreased as we age.[26] Arginine has no side effects and many possible MOJO benefits. However, it should be taken with caution in people with liver or kidney disease.

Last and most important, recent scientific evidence emphasizes the importance of telomeres in healthy aging. Telomeres (end-parts in Greek, so science will continue to astound) are caps on the ends of chromosomes. They have been compared to the plastic ends on shoelaces, which keep the shoestrings from fraying. Telomeres do not participate in genetic expression; they keep the genetic information intact. However, they are worn away as cells divide and when they are sufficiently shortened the cell can no longer divide. Shortened telomeres predict chronic diseases and the disability and mortality they herald.[27] One appears to be as old as their telomeres. The telomere's length can be correlated with the individual cell's biological age. There is a great deal of interest in developing drugs to repair telomeres but there is a natural way to keep telomeres healthy: exercise.

In the Nurses' Health Study, investigators measured 7,800 nurses' telomere lengths. The lengths were not only associated with exercise but correlated with the vigor of the exercise.[28]

An investigation of twins in Britain compared telomere length in white blood cells according to the amount of exercise experienced. This is an especially important study because it specifically looks at environmental influences. Subjects who exercised had less attenuated telomeres. The authors estimated that active exerciser's DNA was on average equivalent to DNA ten years younger than sedentary persons.[29] Exercise of your body and brain is the best antiaging activity known. Get with it!

Chapter 10

Ingestion Suggestion

Your Food Can Save Your Cells

We briefly dealt with the major principles of an antiaging diet in the chapter on recommended lifestyle but overall diet is important to good health. So, this chapter is an enlarged essay on understanding a life-promoting diet.

WHAT EXACTLY DOES DIET MEAN?

Some of the most important inclinations we have in life are determined by what we value and the goals we set to achieve them. Early in our lives, we valued educational goals and then set about to establish meaningful careers. We went through the mate-choosing dance, and expended great amounts of effort raising our families. We grew in the process and helped others. Now in the autumn of our lives, the so-called golden years, our goals have changed. The most important goal now should be to maintain our quality of life to keep the golden years golden. What we ingest has a great deal of influence on our excellence of later health.

"Diet" is an often-mentioned word but rarely in a meaningful way. The word is used habitually as a pejorative implying a dreaded experience. However, concerning our health, it is one of our more important activities. A number of organizations make considerable money managing people's diets. Yet, the average person and even some doctors have very superficial understandings of what makes a diet superior.

Searching for diet books on the Amazon website registers thousands of hits. Many books on a subject indicate there is considerable need for answers and the definitive book does not exist. We continue to concentrate on the principles of health-promoting behaviors; in this chapter we focus on what makes diets healthy. In fact, the majority of scientific literature and much of the not so scientific focus on either regional diets or recommended diets by celebrity dietary authorities, which is important but not as useful as understanding what makes a diet healthy. The most important information is what makes diets health-promoting or not.

The word "diet," which has to be one on the most often-used words in health literature, comes from ancient Greek meaning "a way of life." It has changed to mean what one eats or in some cases avoids eating. Specifically, it denotes adhering to specific foods, at specific times, in specific amounts, or combinations of the three for religious, weight loss, medical, or health reasons. Diets describe consumption of foods and food is fuel for the body.

THE GEOGRAPHIC DIETS

Diets for weight loss abound as the most popular and some indirectly achieve a healthier state through weight loss but for rock-solid dependability; we should trust the two most studied geographically named diets: the Mediterranean diet and the Okinawan diet. Located thousands of miles apart with vastly different cultures, they are *the diets of the longest-lived and healthiest people on earth*. The Mediterranean diet is primarily the diet of southern Italy and people living in the south of Italy live longer than northerners do. Okinawa is a southern Japanese island and the Okinawans live longer than other Japanese. These statistics are particularly impressive when one considers that the Italians (#4) and Japanese (#1) are countries having the highest national longevity on Earth.

The two diets are more similar than different. The main difference is the calories from fat; the Okinawans consume less than one-third of their energy from lipid calories, whereas the Italians consume over 40% of their energy intake from fat. It is notable that the Italian fat derived calories are from unsaturated olive oil. Aside from the unsaturated "good" fats, olive oil has antioxidant substances, which contribute to its health-promoting qualities. We are not going to examine other popular diets such as DASH and the Pritikin diet because they share much in common and are not as well studied as the two diets mentioned.

Foods, making up the diets, deliver energy and nutrients, which provide essential building materials. Energy is essential to supply our life force.

As we all know, food's energy is measured in calories (large and small). A calorie as in common usage, more properly a kilocalorie, is a heat energy measure, the amount necessary to raise a kilogram of water one degree Celsius. Not much, unless multiplied several thousand times, which is what we consume daily. This energy production keeps our body's temperature at about 98.6 degrees F (recently changed to 98.2 degrees F), which varies slightly depending on the site of measurement (mouth, ear, anus, skin). When our metabolism speeds up, to fight an infection, our body's temperature rises, termed a "fever."

THE SCOOP ON ESSENTIAL NUTRIENTS

Our bodies cannot manufacture a number of vital substances, called vitamins. Initially, vitamins were thought to be amino acids, so they were called vital amines. The name change to vitamins resulted from the discovery that they were not all amino acids. There are thirteen vitamins and severe deficiencies result in well-described diseases, such as scurvy. Certain of these vitamins may become deficient in the elderly because of absorption deficiencies, dietary lack, or reduced absorption to the sun. Vitamins that tend to become dietary deficiencies in the elderly include: vitamin D, vitamin B12 (82% of the elderly are deficient in one study), and folic acid.

Vitamin D is the sunshine vitamin for healthy bones. Actually, it supports over three hundred biochemical reactions for bone and muscle health. In an Australian study of independently living elderly (over 70 years) 88% were deficient in vitamin D, which was the highest rate of any vitamin.[1] Deficiency in children (rickets) and in elderly causes a soft bone disorder, which can lead to increased risk of fractures. In adults, deficiency can cause musculoskeletal pain and muscle weakness. Although vitamin D is not excreted by the kidneys (a good safely net), it requires huge doses to become toxic—over 4,000 units a day. In cases of deficiency, supplements can decrease high blood pressure.

Lower vitamin D levels were measured in people with greater cognitive decline in China.[2] Also, a study accessed the rates of mental decline in elderly people over an eight-year period and the vitamin D level was predictive of the rate of decline.[3] In a large well-done study, the Framingham Study, lower vitamin D levels were associated with the development of dementia.[4] The authors point out that this does not ensure that taking vitamin D would prevent dementia.

Active vitamin D is produced by sunlight acting on the skin to convert D2 to D3, so, take the active supplement D3. Taking 1,000 units daily is recommended in people over 65.

Vitamin B12 is the metabolic supervisor of all the cells in the body. It is especially important in brain health. It can increase the energy level. The main problem with B12 is not its intake; it is its absorption. To be absorbed, it needs to combine with a substance secreted by the stomach—intrinsic factor. B12 also needs acid for optimal absorption. The aging lining of the stomach sometimes produces less of each of these necessary substances, ergo, a deficiency results. Since the problem is absorption, oral supplements may not correct the problem; B12 is given by injection or under the tongue (sublingual).

Folic acid or its salt, folate, is a B vitamin that is deficient in 40% of elderly people.[5] Deficiency is more often seen in persons with high blood pressure. Folate is a brain vitamin and deficiencies might be considered to contribute to dementias of the elderly but studies have not shown an association. All three of the vitamins mentioned can easily be taken as supplements.

In addition, our bodies cannot make nine amino acids and two fatty acids, which are necessary, but a normal diet usually provides adequate supplies. One can be assured of adequacy by eating a balanced diet. Long-standing special diets, such as vegan, run a risk of vitamin deficiencies, especially B12.

Understanding what specifically makes diets health-promoting is all important. It is not optimal to know which foods are healthy; we must know *what makes foods health-promoting.* We individually have differing tastes and eat accordingly. Knowing how to tweak our chosen diets seems more desirable than changing over; behavioral compliance usually depends on the extent of change and success depends on the extent of compliance. Principles allow preference in changes made. We will explore several recently popularized concepts concerning healthy dieting: total caloric intake and nutritional density of various foods. We will revisit two of the more important nutritional concepts, which are established but largely unappreciated: glycemic index and glycemic load. Concerning remaining well, especially as you get older, these are two of the most important considerations.

Foods can be said to be health-promoting or not depending on what they contain that can be absorbed. Among the major minerals (termed "electrolytes" because they have electrical charges), the amount of sodium we consume is in the news recently. Potassium, another key beneficial mineral, is rarely mentioned. Although natural diets provide enough minerals and our bodies can withhold or excrete them to compensate to a certain extent, adjustments of processed foods, fast foods, and other modern alterations can override our natural defenses. The Third National Health and Nutrition Examination Survey calculated the sodium/potassium dietary ratios of over 12,000 subjects, finding that lower intakes of sodium and higher intakes of potassium were associated with a 46% reduction in mortality over 14.8 years of follow-up.[6] Wow, we survive according to what we eat.

What we consume matters. Processed foods often contain huge amounts of sodium and this can be seen on the nutritional facts labels, which will help you choose more healthful products. Processed foods sell better because people crave salt. Salt was hard to come by in prehistoric times. It is essential in maintaining hydration. In excess, it retains excess fluid, resulting in hypertension.

AGING'S DAMAGE AND FOOD

Aging, after all, is the result of living. Biochemical energy production in cells produces damage from the by-product of free radicals. Diet influences aging and chronic disease development by avoiding excess disorderly free radicals from producing a state termed "oxidative stress." Oxidative stress is when excess free radicals are produced in our cells faster than our defense mechanisms can neutralize them, causing damage. Oxidative stress can result from a big meal, sporadic exercise, or release of stress hormones from worry. Oxidative stress levels determine the rate of damage our cells endure as we age. Aging is the damage our cells get from living. Neutralization of damage is from antioxidants. Dietary intake can improve health status by decreasing the harmful elements (free radicals) or increasing the beneficial elements (antioxidants).

Animal cells, unlike plant cells, do not directly produce energy-yielding substances. Thus, our bodies absorb and process energy-retaining substances from plants and other animals. Life requires that cellular energy be produced through oxidative "burning" which releases "sparks" (free radicals) that are potentially harmful.

A higher caloric content of the diet produces more "sparks" for the body to contend. As a first line of protection, caloric restriction reduces the amount of "sparks" generated. Abundant research shows caloric restriction in various experimental animals, including non-human primates, extends lifespans.

Caloric restriction is reducing the caloric intake by 10% to 30% of what animals eat when allowed to eat freely. This is not such that malnutrition results. Many scientists regard reductions in caloric consumption to be the single greatest extender of longevity; it can double the useful lifespan in many studies. Thirty percent caloric restriction in various non-human primates significantly reduces chronic diseases including heart disease, stroke, and diabetes.[7]

Our bodies are alive because of energy produced by chemical "fires" in our bodies' cells and similar to regular real fires we can see, the amount of fuel burned overall determines the amount of sparks (free radicals) produced but the amount of heat produced by different fuels is important as well. Of course, eating more glucose-laden food allows more glucose to be absorbed. As the blood glucose rises, the body reacts by secreting more insulin, which stuffs the glucose into cells, just as if stoking a fire. Mice when fed a high-sugar diet developed more damage from oxidants.[8] It is reasonable to conclude that the same applies to humans.

The more intense the cellular energy production, the more sparks are created. It's not just the total intake of calories that produces more sparks. Foods release glucose at different rates causing our blood glucose to rise at different rates. Damage caused by sparks depends on the number of sparks produced which can overwhelm the body's defenses.

Thus, foods are healthful or not depend both on the amount and rapidity they cause the blood glucose to increase. Foods have their specific rates of producing high or low levels of glucose after consumption determined by absorption rates and it is termed the glycemic index (GI for short). The GI is from 0 to 100, with 100 being the highest because it has the highest rate for consumption of pure glucose. Numbers above 70 are considered high and below 50 are considered low or safer. Remember low is slow.

Markers for free radicals increased in people who ate higher GI foods.[9] Slower sugar absorption is desirable because elevated blood sugar is forced into cells and processed in cellular furnaces at a more rapid rate. Markers for greater risk for heart attacks and stroke are increased in people with higher GI diets.[10] In the PREDIMED study, thousands of elderly community-dwelling subjects' GI and GLs (glucose loads) were determined. Those with high GI diets had double the mortality rate.[11] Therefore, not just the amount of food but the kind of foods we eat matters. It is wise to keep track of the high GI foods, such as watermelon, and consume smaller amounts at each meal and to arrange your diet to include more low GI foods, which you enjoy. There is some evidence for the detrimental effect of large sugar-laden sodas.

MINERALS ARE IMPORTANT AS WELL

It's not only what we consider is in the food, designations such as meat, fruits, and vegetables don't tell the whole story. The devil is also in the details. Minerals we consume are vital. There are at least twenty-two necessary minerals in the human body. Eight are the major minerals and fourteen are termed "trace" minerals because of their small amounts. Among the major minerals (called electrolytes in medicine), seven are regularly measured by blood tests. Minerals, except for heavy metals, are easily eliminated by the kidneys which have exquisitely sensitive processes to keep the concentrations within narrow limits. People with kidney disease must be careful about mineral intake.

Sodium is an important mineral related to health. Sodium is the main atom in table salt. In the middle ages it was more valuable than gold. It is a desirable condiment to season food and is necessary for life by keeping the body's water intact. The more salt ingested, the more water retained. Thus, salt is bad for hypertensives.

Potassium is a vital mineral contained mostly within our cells (97% is in cells). CDC recommends a daily intake of almost 5 grams, about double that of sodium. Deficiencies of potassium are dangerous because it is what makes the heart beat normally. Additional potassium is usually prescribed when diuretics are given. Ironically, potassium injections are used for criminal executions. But it would be difficult to take enough with normal kidney function to pose a problem.

Magnesium is another important mineral, which helps regulate hundreds of biochemical reactions to keep bones and muscles healthy. Almost two-thirds of older adults eat diets lower in magnesium than recommended. People with low magnesium intake have increased risk of developing cardiovascular disease.[12] A magnesium supplement in older people with normal kidney function is a good idea. Magnesium is connected to energy production in muscle and connected to the rate of aging through the reduction of cell damage.[13]

ATOMIC FIRE EXTINGUISHERS

Antioxidants are "spark" extinguishers that neutralize "sparks" produced from metabolism; they are both produced by the body and are taken in in the diet. The antioxidant content of food is probably the most important factor promoting health. Certain foods such as tomatoes that are loaded with antioxidants are beneficial. An Italian study of more than 5,000 participants showed that cancer of the esophagus and stomach were reduced by a greater intake of tomatoes.[14] Tomatoes are reasonable examples of important pillars of the healthy diets such as the Mediterranean and Okinawan diets. We are all aware of the famous yummy Italian tomato sauces. Both diets consume fruits and vegetables regularly.

Both diets are hearty regarding legumes (beans, peas, lentils, and others less common). Legumes, not a common food in America (I asked some people who did not know the word), have the highest antioxidants of any food. Another staple of the Okinawan diet is the sweet potato, which is loaded with nutritional content and antioxidants, perhaps balancing the relatively unhealthy (high glycemic index) white rice they consume. Brown rice is healthier. Both cultures consume low glycolytic index grains, Okinawans more than Mediterranean dieters.

Likewise, sources of protein are typically fish and seafood in Italy and pork in Okinawa but pork is eaten meagerly in Okinawa, usually at monthly festivals. Both diets consume fatty or red meats very sparingly. Okinawans have a unique tendency, I want to mention again, cited in the Blue Zones book, of avoiding stuffing themselves. They stop eating when they are about 80% full. I started applying this concept about a year ago and lost (keeping off) 10 pounds. I am satisfied with half of a large-serving restaurant portion. I get two meals for the price of one.

The key to these two billboard famous diets is the antioxidant content and the avoidance of gorging with carbohydrates. Keeping the harmful products of metabolism under control is crucial to the antiaging process. The rapidity with which we age determines how fast we are wearing out and the extent of wearing out determines how fast we will get chronic diseases.

A side benefit that should be of interest to well-balanced men is that the unfortunate ED is improved by the amount of antioxidant foods consumed. In a Canadian study of 1,200 diabetic men the percentage with ED dropped significantly with consumption of fruits and vegetables.[15] Esposito studied 95 men placed on the Mediterranean diet compared to a group not on it for two years, and found that men on the Mediterranean diet were three times more likely not to have ED.[16] Similar dietary changes in women had sexuality benefits.[17]

In several European studies dietary changes improved mental function. In the PREDIMED-NAVARRA study, Mediterranean diets supplemented with olive oil or nuts significantly improved cognition in people over 70 years.[18] Another excellently crafted study, done in Manhattan, noted a protective effect from developing Alzheimer's disease by ingesting some of the foods consumed in the geographic healthy diets.[19] They noted: "The results of the current study indicate that higher consumption of certain foods (olive oil salad dressing, nuts, fish, tomatoes, poultry, cruciferous vegetables (cauliflower, cabbage, garden cress, bok choy, broccoli, brussel sprouts), fruits, dark and green leafy vegetables) and lower of other foods (high-fat dairy, red meat, organ meats, and butter) may be associated with a decreased risk of developing Alzheimer's Disease."

An attention-grabbing study, published this year, compared MRI brain scans of subjects in their 50s and 60s, separating them into high and low Mediterranean diet groups.[20] None of the participants were having cognitive difficulties at the beginning of the study. After five years, the low Mediterranean diet subjects had anatomical loss of brain tissue in vital areas, whereas the high Mediterranean diet adherents retained brain substance. Adjusting one's diet does not just provide a longer life; it is scientifically shown to maintain the quality of life.

The vitamin and supplement industry manufactures most of the well-known antioxidants for consumption but for some unexplained reason, natural dietary consumption is superior and some supplements are not helpful. Research over time on large population groups conclude some antioxidant supplements may be harmful. Excess beta-carotene, and vitamins A and E may increase mortality.[21]

The majority of diets focus on weight control and weight control is important, but eating a healthy diet is much more vital and will control weight as well. The principles of a health-promoting diet include emphasizing antioxidant and nutrient rich foods (avoiding processed foods), including fiber, eating the right fats and avoiding the bad fats, and consuming moderate amounts of wine.

In summary, we age by the process of living through oxidizing food, mainly sugar. This generates substances that damage our cells (free radicals). When more free radicals are produced than our bodies can neutralize, it is termed "oxidative stress" and aging accelerates. Diet, as mentioned, has two healthful purposes. First, diet needs to supply nutrients necessary for healthy living. These include minerals, vitamins, and other essentials. Next, diet can be designed to reduce production of harmful substances and to consume substances which neutralize the harmful substances our bodies produce.

Chapter 11

Get Out

The Health Benefits of an Optimized Social Life

WHAT IS SOCIALIZATION AND WHY DID IT COME ABOUT?

Humans are undoubtedly the most social creatures on the planet. After the incredible closeness of a nine-month gestational period, humans yearn for friendships from the time of birth. Socialization begins in infancy and is a profound instructor that forms the human personality. Socialization is necessary to form a tribe. And why is it necessary to form a tribe? Among major predators, humans have the least natural bodily weaponry and physical agility. They made up for their defects and became the greatest and certainly the most lethal species by using special skills and by pack-hunting. Gifted with upright posture and grasping hands, pack-hunting prehistoric humans could launch multiple projectiles and bring down animals much larger than themselves. Survival required tribal living, which required socialization.

Throughout history, those who launched projectiles more accurately were valued. Today the emphasis remains: quarterbacks, pitchers, and point guards are the celebrated athletic stars because they can throw objects more accurately. Star throwers need a team as well, and teams' names are suggestive of tribes; consider the Redskins, Indians, Chiefs, Braves, and Hawks (formerly Blackhawks). Society values skills long after their time has passed because ancient values are woven into their ethos. When some societal trait seems out of place, it's from evolution.

Early in the tribal process, religious rites became part of the socialization process, according to anthropologists, more than scores of centuries ago. Religion consolidated authority, sanctified war, provided sources of food, and assured an afterlife. Religion was perhaps the keystone of socialization, as we will discuss later.

I have arrived at a personal conclusion of the most important of human attainments; what we all, often subconsciously, strive to attain—meaning. According to Professor Robert Nozick, from Harvard, one of the great modern philosophers, meaning by definition requires crossing boundaries of other sentient beings (i.e., involving others). Love is generally considered the most important attainment but it is but a subset of achieving meaning and "love" that is without meaning is a worthless endeavor. A person can care enough for another to say they love them, but the importance of "love" as Spinoza opined depends on meaning being given to the loving one.

The *Mona Lisa* when placed in a bank vault remains valuable but forfeits meaning. Happiness also is frequently considered the highest human goal, by utilitarian philosophy, but happiness devoid of meaning, for instance taking drugs, is shallow indeed. Thus, meaning is the result of social interaction. Meaning is subjective and science requires objectivity. Thus, social scientists study social integration, which is examining the way we search for meaning!

MICRO-SOCIALIZATION IS VERY IMPORTANT

I divide socialization into macro-socialization and micro-socialization. Macro-socialization is one's acquaintances in general, the big picture. Micro-socialization includes the most important and closest people in your life, a select group. "One," a hit song by Three Dog Night in 1969, opens with the line "one is the loneliest number." By all the scientific data, the song is accurate. Recent multiple well-done studies have shown social integration has a significant benefit on health. Marriages, cohabitation, numbers of social contacts, trust in social contacts, social group contacts, and religiosity are all significant. In the Swedish Kungsholmen project being socially integrated lengthened useful life even in those over 75 years of age.[1] In a subset of the Kungsholmen study, over 1,200 elderly subjects who had good mental function when the study began, 14% developed dementia. Establishing a good social network reduces the chance of the dreaded dementia by 60%.[2] Socialization deposits cash in your mental bank.

Marriage is the most important human social relationship. If social integration is an important determinant of our healthy longevity, marriage should influence our health and longevity. The data clearly shows that men who married live longer than those who did not. A vast study of American men (67,000) showed significant health benefits of being happily married.[3]

The never married fared the worst in all age groups and married but separated were next.

Further and more interesting, marital benefits are evident on a molecular level. Telomeres (telo = end, meres = substance) are the important ends of our chromosomes, serving to protect our DNA's integrity. Scientists can measure the length of our telomeres and determine our "cellular" age. Cells examined in middle-aged married adults were compared to those who were widowed, divorced, separated, or never married and married people's cells were significantly younger.[4] In another important study, telomere length and the concentration of an enzyme which breaks down telomeres (increased bad, decreased good) was measured.[5] Telomere shortening and the destructive enzyme were increased in subjects with reduced social support. They also had lower optimism, and higher hostility. Thus, our cells, reflecting the biochemical aging process, are younger with optimized socialization.

In addition, like many aspects of behavior on health, the benefit also equates with the quality of the marriage experience. Health of marital partners varies depending whether the relationship is positive or negative.[6] Husbands lived longer when considered a confidant providing emotional support by their wife. Psychological closeness and trust were the important shared beneficial characteristics. The British Household Panel Survey examined social relationships including the satisfaction from work environment and similarly found the quality of the social experiences determined derived satisfaction.[7] Aren't those simply features of obtaining a meaningful life?

And you are in control by the actions you take. Just apply the golden rule to your life partner. Treat them in the manner that you want to be treated. Complement often, appreciate often, and understand more often. Ask for explanations when in doubt. Make understanding and communication the pillars of your relationship and you will both benefit.

Nuances of marital relationships surprise by significantly impacting health. Health of elderly mothers varied whether they had stepchildren versus biological children; those who raised stepchildren became disabled more often as they aged and required institutionalization sooner.[8] In addition, fathers raising stepchildren, on the other hand, died sooner than those who raised biological children. Nuances of life's important experiences continue to amaze.

RELIGIOUS SOCIALIZATION'S EFFECTS

In large studies of religious denominations, Mormons, Seventh Day Adventists, and Jews experience reduced mortality rates when compared to the general population in the United States.[9] Medical care has improved considerably and often is credited with better national health. In a large study of older Amish subjects, however, who are known to use minimal amounts of medical care, their longevity was significantly better than non-Amish.[10] Amish are allowed tobacco and alcohol; they do not eat a low fat diet. They work hard and, as we all know, avoid most technology advances; preferring the simple life. What they excel in is social integration; their lives are very socially integrated, arguably the most emphasized in America. They help each other build houses and make repairs as needed. Their lives are a natural affirmation of the value of social integration.

Environmental factors like disciplined lifestyles, dietary restrictions, and discrete gene pools may provide conventional explanations for such findings. Some intriguing data, nevertheless, originated from using the frequency of attendance at religious services as a presumed indicator of religiosity.[9] These studies have examined correlations between religiosity (yes, it's a word) and health status. Religious attendance is independently associated with decreased mortality when other factors known to influence survival positively are mathematically excluded.

In one large study conducted across three decades, infrequent attendees at religious services with similar health habits and prior good health status had higher rates of mortality from circulatory, digestive, and respiratory conditions. In another study with a 28-year follow-up, frequent attendees at religious services had 36% lower mortality rates than occasional or non-attendees, but they also smoked less, exercised more, and socialized more frequently. When their healthier lifestyles' effects on mortality were mathematically excluded, the frequent attendees still retained a 23% reduction in mortality. Believe it.

In 1992, Bryant reported that mortality among African Americans who did not attend religious services was twice that of weekly attendees.[11] In a smaller study that estimated religiosity using variables other than service attendance, little improvement in overall lifestyle was found, but elsewhere the same investigators noted that Protestant males are more overweight but smoke less. It appears that religiosity as measured by frequency of attending formal religious services may or may not promote healthier behaviors, but has an added health advantage not explained by conventional associated factors.

Regardless of data from multiple studies on health benefits from attending church, that criterion remains suspect as a proxy for religion. After all, religious services have many different meanings rather than the extent of faith-based beliefs. Perhaps regularly attending rock concerts ensures similar benefits; after all, perhaps an hour of mental involvement is the benefactor. Private religious activities, however, including prayer, meditation, or Bible study, not just attending religious services, in almost four thousand older adults had significant survival benefits.[12] This benefit disappeared in those who were disabled. The authors suggest that *for maximum benefits commence spiritual activity before disability.* In addition, how people rated their intrinsic spiritual beliefs was beneficial in their hospitalized outcomes.[13] Hospitalized patients who were transcendent in their faith in God had better results when treated for the same diseases.

I realized this in my practice of heart surgery for over three decades; the last question I asked patients when giving informed consent before surgery was: "How are you with the lord?" Only a handful out of thousands objected to the question. If they did not have a religious contact, I asked that they have a visit from the chaplain; to those who told me they did not need a visit from the chaplain, I responded: It's not for you, it's for me. I also stopped by my church to pray early each morning before major cases. The pastor kept the rear door to the sanctuary unlocked for me. My operative results are among the best in the world literature.

Do I believe God intervenes directly in daily life—probably not—but believing you have covered all bases surely works. In dealing once with a deeply religious person who was conflicted because of legitimate beliefs as to whether to rely on God or medicine to fix her heart valve, we sat and talked. I have no doubt that God could fix your heart, I noted, and you seem to be worthy, but God for some reason does not seem to be in that business. He has allowed believers like me, over the past three thousand years, members of all faiths, to work out techniques to accomplish that task. Her valve was successfully fixed without compromising her religious values.

Resilience is a personality characteristic that strongly promotes longevity.[14] Being able to roll with the punches of life is important in reducing the harmful stress life imposes. Some of the unhappiest people I have encountered are those who believe life has been unfair to them; life is a stage, a medium for us to act our parts and at best learn. To expect rewards and punishments in harmony with how good or bad we consider our behavior is absurd. As Shakespeare had Hamlet so ably observe, "For there is nothing either good or bad, but thinking makes it so."

Religion helps build resilience, which may be its mechanism for improving health.[15] Believing in a personal supreme being gives comfort and reverses the notion of a meaningless universe. I don't play golf but golf is a good metaphor for the problems life presents us. Life has sand traps, which even the most skilled golfers cannot avoid. The actual skill of living, like the best golfers, is to not only recognize the traps and try to avoid them, but moreover, be able to get out when getting in the traps inevitably happens. Religious and social networking provides support, enhancing coping mechanisms—ergo resilience.

Patients who are ill have been found to suffer significantly higher mortality if, by their report, they are psychologically engaged in a "religious struggle" involving uncertainties about their relationship with God.[16] Asking why did this happen to me is a pointless exercise.

Secular socialization's influence on health is much less studied but when a subject of inquiry, is also is proven to reduce mortality. In one scientific trial, the health benefits increased as the number of regular social contacts increased. The Third National Health and Nutrition Examination Survey measured inflammatory markers that measured risk for heart attacks and stroke in 14,000 subjects according to their social integration.[17] The scientists created a social network index using information about marital status; number of contacts with family, friends, and neighbors; frequency of religious service attendance; and participation in voluntary organizations. In the elderly men, dangerous markers indicating health risk almost doubled in those with few social contacts.

Elderly community-dwelling adults were asked to rate the success of their aging process and among other criteria, the number of close friends correlated with more successful estimates of their aging.[18] They aged better as the number of close friends rose. Starting social integration, even in the elderly, enriches well-being.[19] Long-term nursing home residents were invited to join social clubs. Personal identity strength, cognitive ability, and well-being were measured at the commencement of the intervention and 12 weeks later. Well-being according to a number of parameters increased from this brief social club participation. Get involved whatever your situation.

As a general principle of living's influence on health, chronic disease problems are incremental, slowly building over decades. Each cigarette inflicts a minuscule bit of damage and social factors likewise are similar. Tiny bits of more meaningful social experiences reduce the wear and tear of aging. Increasing socializing is straightforward. One simply finds more activities that are social and participates. But social integration is more than amount of time spent with others. As seen earlier from a number of studies the satisfaction quality experience gives is paramount and more complex. To explore this, I must engage an area where I have minimal applicable professional training—psychology of relationships. Sincerely connecting with people is the start of a more rewarding social integration.

GROWING PEOPLE SKILLS

People skills are important, rarely considered, behaviors because they often are taken for granted. An excellent test (albeit for work people skills but can be applied generally) is found at the website: http://www.mindtools.com/pages/article/newTMM_36.htm. Take the test and evaluate whether you should grow in people skills. All of us can grow. People skills can add more meaning to our lives.

Appreciation of those you surround yourself with is important. How many of us wish we had voiced more appreciation to those departed we care for more often? Don't continue that mistake; actively appreciate your friends and loved ones, especially those you have chosen as partners in life. Genuine appreciation is a coin of great value with two sides—contentment for the recipient and giver as well. Like an echo, kind words come back. The Bible instructs, "A man that hath friends must shew himself friendly" (Prov. 18:24). Attentiveness, responsive, approachable, outgoing, and social are synonyms of friendly. Friendly constantly rewards.

Appreciation must be sincere. Place yourself into fortunate mental mode when evaluating friends and loved ones. Those you associate with must have some good attributes or you wouldn't find them of interest. I am fortunate my friends and loved ones are smart, creative, and talented; I am fortunate indeed. Surround yourself with friends you can appreciate and you will find it easy to appreciate. Appreciation is directed gratitude.

If you want to be liked by others, till your relationship's soil with kindness. Kindnesses are especially effective when they are a surprise. Every once in a while, when I am down, I drive to Starbucks, order a double expresso, and hand an extra $10 for the next patron's coffee. My mood elevates from just imagining how that simple gesture makes someone else feel. Unanticipated kindnesses are even more rewarding when given to a friend.

Don't gossip. Gossip, by definition, is about the personal matters, rumor or fact, about details of other people's lives, often malicious. The gossiper's incentive is that the gossiped about would prefer the information being disclosed to remain secret. When I had supervisory roles and was told morsels of gossip, I had a single criterion as to its worth: I asked, "Would you mind if I ask so and so about this?" If they replied no, I dismissed the matter. About 90% of the gossip was summarily dismissed, thereby.

Remove the control motivation from those that are important to your life. We are classified as a species Homo sapiens (wise man), which is mostly true but competitive man would be more accurate. Often our worth, especially at work, is determined by comparing how well or how efficiently we do a task.

The overwhelming interest we have in sports emphasizes such a fixation. Aside from sports, overt competition is often more detrimental than beneficial; it has no place between your closest relatives and friends.

Deliberate and integrate your life strategies with your closest persons so they will understand and support your actions. Sharing your life's hopes and dreams with those who care, will as much as anything promote positive bonding and future understanding and support.

Among all most important human skill sets , the least mastered is listening. Workers in mental health professions train for years in dynamic listening. I have run across few people who have listened so well that I felt for a brief moment that they thought what I had to say was the most important discourse in the world. One master listener was Dr. Harold Cummings, Dean of Admissions at Tulane University Medical School. He was an elfin man with frayed lab coat cuffs, usually no tie, oversized head, and ever-present pipe, but he always relocated from behind a huge desk and arranged a chair facing you, barely a foot apart, and you became exalted. Later, Yoda in the Star Wars series reminded me of him, without the pointy ears. We should all endeavor to be better listeners. We would bestow good will, strengthen our social integration, and learn more by doing so.

Emotions are generally considered as characteristics opposing reason. Greek philosophy, the Bible, and modern philosophy all recommend that emotions be controlled. Emotions filter our factual input by personalizing ideas. There is survival value in emotions. Imagine the different response of a prehistoric when at night hearing a growling saber-toothed tiger. The response would vary whether it was just outside the cave, at the periphery of the tribe, or across the river at the campsite of a warring tribe. We no longer hear saber-toothed tigers at night.

Anger is a primitive protective mechanism instilled in all advanced creatures. It is primarily territorial with an original "you have violated my geographic boundaries" connotation but more often now, the violation is regarding psychological boundaries. Anger provokes powerful hormonal responses, preparing the body for flight or fight responses if used wrongly. Wrong use is termed "fury," "frenzy," or "rage." Displaying annoyance or irritation is all right but not to be used too often. Used inappropriately, anger is arguably the most harmful emotional and social response we can muster up.

Anger was a survival mechanism in ancient times but is rarely needed in the modern world. It is a great impersonator; the angry person strongly believes they are seeing the world correctly, when they may be wrong and the certainty of being wronged predisposes to overreaction. How many times is an anger burst responsible for a serious mistake—even a criminal act? When I was boxing, we were coached not to get angry when peeved, and having someone hit your face repeatedly is anger-provoking for sure. But an angry boxer would mindlessly flail about, forgetting the principles and rules of boxing. Uncontrolled anger leads to a number of situations that are mostly regrettable after its dissipation: road rage, senseless violence, and hurtful statements from deep within the Freudian id.

Prominent psychologists opine anger has underlying flashpoints that we should search for to control anger. With few pathological exceptions, anger can be controlled. Why am I getting upset is a very good question to ask; it brings rationality, which confronts irrationality. Jewish friends, during trying moments, would say, "This too shall pass." Also, remember what Dr. Richard Carlson has to say in his book *Don't Sweat the Small Stuff . . . And It's All Small Stuff*—he includes advice such as "Choose your battles wisely"; "Remind yourself that when you die, your 'in' box won't be empty"; and "Make peace with imperfection." All great ideas.

Sometimes, especially in marriage, spouses are critical of one another, which can develop into adopting roles. One person tends to be more critical and demanding, while the other tends to withdraw or shut down in response to conflict. Douglas Tilley, a proponent of emotion-focused therapy, notes that 85% of the time men tend to be the withdrawer. The reason may be biological—men's cardiovascular systems are more responsive to stress, so tuning out your mate is an attempt to avoid uncomfortable sensations.

To break the negative pattern of conflict in your relationship, next time things get heated, let your partner know what's going on with you by saying: "I can see this issue is important to you. I'm feeling too angry to discuss it right now, though, so let's come back to it once we've cooled off." A caution, when using this valuable approach: go back to deal with the issue, when the situation has cooled down or this problem solving method will fail.

Fix recurring problems, especially those that call up painful emotions. Take advice from one of the smartest people of history, Albert Einstein, who is credited with saying: "Insanity is doing the same thing over and over again and expecting different results." It is wise to determine what is important and repetitive and deal with it.

To stop this trouble from ruining your relationship, you'll need to address the bigger issues underlying your difficulty. Take turns discussing with your partner what this loaded issue really means to you. When your partner is talking, your job is to listen, be nonjudgmental, and to find something in their perspective that makes sense to you. When it's your turn to talk, they should be doing the same thing. By treading more gently into touchy areas, you should at least be able to agree to disagree or make some small concessions for one another. Over time even small concessions add up.

Kato studied the personality characteristics of centenarians and found they were optimistic, outgoing (socially integrating), and freely expressed (not holding internally) emotions.[20] This indicates that a positive attitude toward life goes a long way toward lengthening lifespan. This is accomplished by slowing the aging process. Applaud the good life, which we can all achieve and which, if we work at it, can make it better.

Chapter 12

The Essentials about
Essential Hypertension

Hypertension is truly the silent killer. In over 90% of cases of hypertension the cause is unknown to medical science—surprisingly, called essential hypertension, thus the title of the chapter. It is the most common chronic disease accelerator in people over 65 years of age. Hypertension pushes the gas petal for damage to arteries; it is reckless driving for the arteries. Everyone knows high blood pressure can be harmful but actions to manage it properly are not generally appreciated.

Overall, one of three adults has hypertension; this climbs to two of three in those over 65 years of age. Twenty percent of hypertensives do not know they have a problem and about 40% with hypertension are not being treated.[1] More alarming is the fact that even though highly effective treatment is available, only one-third of hypertension is adequately controlled medically.[2]

Adequately controlled blood pressure means maintaining a blood pressure below 140/90. The top figure is the pulse resulting from a heartbeat and the bottom value is pressure between beats. This must be a resting measurement, preferably sitting quietly for a few minutes before measurement.

Recently, the recommendations are out raising the allowable blood pressure in people over 60 years of age. As a scientist working in the field, it does not make sense that older means reducing the treatment standards. If anything since older people have more vascular disease and less reserve, treatment should probably be intensified. The American Heart Association, which has no political allegiances and lots of expertise, agrees that the standard of lowering blood pressure below 140/90 mmHg should continue to be the treatment goal.

Hypertension is widely known to increase vascular disease, especially strokes. Just as bad, hypertension is a major contributor to dementia, especially the dreaded Alzheimer's disease.[3] Since there are no effective treatments for Alzheimer's disease and strokes can be devastating, prevention is the only strategy.

Such dismal results in treating hypertension indicate something is wrong with the process of therapy for hypertension. Actually, hypertension's suboptimal management is a superb example of why patient participation in personal health maintenance is necessary. And why basic health knowledge is essential to adequately participate.

The majority of all adults, especially hypertensive adults, are confident that an occasional trip to their doctor is sufficient. The doc is just the coach in your medical care, especially regarding hypertension. The patient is the main determinant of results in outpatient care. Without knowledge of what is going on and what should take place, hypertensives are without checks on their therapy.

A number of effective classes of medicines are available. Medications can be switched when not working and often are combined with other meds to achieve desired results. One answer is the prescribing physician may not have sufficient knowledge as to which meds to use in a particular case.

But the much more common problem is inadequate monitoring and follow-up. Sporadic medical appointments provide only snapshots of what is a dynamic healthiness problem. Blood pressure varies according to the activity, mental state, and time of day. Usually, a single blood pressure recording each visit is used to determine therapy and unless the pressure is markedly elevated, follow-up recordings with reevaluation are usually repeated in weeks or months. Scheduling spacing is not the fault of the doc; scheduling patients weekly, which is how blood pressure needs monitoring, is costly. Thus, patients need to monitor their individual blood pressures.

Let's examine the essentials for improved hypertension therapy. The purpose of the chapter in brief is: first, the circulatory system is an amazing bio-engineering feat formed early in embryonic development. Tiny capillary blood vessels can be found everywhere in the body except for the corneas. Looking at living tissue under a microscope, one observes frantic-appearing red blood cells moving rapidly along little transparent tunnels—releasing their life-giving oxygen and picking up wastes of metabolism. They are both pizza deliverers and garbage collectors. Estimates of the total length of blood vessels in an adult are upwards of 15,000 miles; most are tiny. Placed end to end the vessels from a single person would stretch five and a half times across the United States. Wow!

Blood needs to move from the heart to the lungs, then once filled with oxygen to the tissues, back to the heart, to the lungs, and back to the heart every minute or less (depending on physical activity) and this requires energy from the pumping heart. If our heart were to stop, we would lose consciousness within seconds and be irreversibly dead in about five minutes. The blood pressure that is of concern is on the arterial side, the place where blood is going from the heart to the body. Veins are low pressure and their problems are clots which are obstructions to flow, especially in the legs.

Larger artery's walls (not hardened) are about an eighth of an inch thick and have a lot of elastic fibers for expansion during pulsation when the heart beats. Each heartbeat produces a wave, much like the ocean, that travels from the larger to the smaller arteries. The pulse is sensed by feeling these waves in middle-sized arteries, as a pulse—usually in the wrist. One obviously has pulses all over the body but they are best felt in the wrist, neck, and groin where arteries are superficial.

This vascular system's pressure (your blood pressure) depends on four things: (1) the amount of blood (the average adult male has five liters, roughly five quarts); (2) the ease of runoff of the smaller end arteries; (3) the give of the arteries (i.e., how elastic they are); and (4) how hard the heart pumps.

Overfilling the system is a known cause of high blood pressure. Salt keeps water in the body and in excess overfills the system. If you drink a quart of pure water, your kidneys will excrete the excess within an hour. Lace the water with 1% salt and it will take a day for the kidneys to excrete the excess. Water flows easily out of the kidneys but salt takes kidney energy to excrete making it linger.

The number of regulatory mechanisms of the body exceeds those of our government. Our bodies operate within narrow limits which must rapidly alter depending on conditions. Numerous receptors keep control of the blood pressure through nerves and hormones. The microscopic arteries have muscle that regulates blood flow by constricting or relaxing depending on nerve impulses and hormone concentrations.

Among the many survival mechanisms in our body that are engineering masterpieces is the kidney's ability to control the blood pressure by releasing substances to constrict the small arteries. The kidneys demand the greatest blood flow per weight of any organ, even the brain, because a relatively small amount of waste is cleared from the blood, each passing through the kidneys. If the blood pressure becomes insufficient, death would result; so, kidneys mandate the blood flow is adequate by raising pressure. Secretions from the kidneys to raise blood pressure can cause hypertension and several classes of drugs lower pressure by interfering with the kidney's secretions.

The loss of ease of expansion of our arteries in a pulsatile system would exacerbate pressure with hardening of the arteries. As we age our elastic fibers decrease, as evident in the skin, especially of the face. Faces sag but arteries uncooperatively don't relax to allow lower pressures. The heart pumps the same or even less as we age which is not a causative agent of increasing blood pressure.

The classic criteria for diagnosis of hypertension is having blood pressure over 140/90 recorded multiple times. Two pressures are recorded because our pressures are pulsatile. The higher pressure is termed "systolic," indicating the pressure generated by a heartbeat, and the lesser pressure, termed "diastolic," is the pressure when the heart is filling with blood. The systolic pressure, since long-term damage is mechanical in nature, is the most important to control for health.

A visit to the doctor's office should include a measurement of the blood pressure but is insufficient. The blood pressure varies tremendously according to posture, physical status, mental state, and time of day. The pressure should be taken by a trained person after the patient sits relaxed for at least five minutes in a quiet room. Going to the doctor can be stressful and result in what is termed "white coat hypertension." The staff can be rushed and take pressures too rapidly which can be falsely low.

Those having hypertension and those over 65 should periodically take their pressures at home. There are accurate automatic blood pressure monitors available for less than $100 and are good investments. CVS advanced and Omron 10 series are machines that are highly regarded and recommended. I use an older Omron model for monitoring pressure and have tested its precision with a calibrated manual blood pressure machine (sphygmomanometer) repeatedly, finding it accurate. Your physician can help you check your monitor's accurateness. At least once a year take your blood pressure monitor to your doctor's office and compare the pressures. This will assure you are relying on an accurate instrument.

At a regular time each week, apart from stressful activities, in the middle of the day (blood pressure tends downward in the evening), sit quietly for five minutes and then take your blood pressure, several times. Do not measure pressure just after physical exertion or drinking caffeinated beverages.

Several times each year, measure your blood pressure in both arms. A difference of 10 mm or more may indicate disease in the arteries supplying the arms.

Home monitoring will promote control superior to relying on the doctor and much cheaper. This is because over time meds need to change as the body changes. When changes in meds are necessary, remember: Most blood pressure meds take several weeks to exert an influence. Some take six weeks to fully influence pressures.

Hypertension is generally classed as primary (essential) or secondary. Ninety-five percent is primary because no specific cause can be found. In medicine, hypertension without an identifiable cause is termed "essential." I'm not sure whether essential is the most descriptive modifier, except that it is essential that it is treated properly.

Secondary hypertension means there is an underlying other disease causing the elevated blood pressure that needs to be treated to reduce the elevation. Hypertension developing early or being difficult to treat needs to be evaluated for other diseases.

Unless pressures are very high (i.e., more than 160/90), a trial of lifestyle modification initially can be tried. Numerous studies have shown reductions in pressure by weight reduction, dietary changes, regular physical activity, and moderation in alcohol consumption. Weight reduction and dietary changes are the most efficient with up to a 20 mm drop in systolic pressures.[1]

Almost a half century ago a landmark paper examined the root cause of how blood pressure increases as we age. The Cook Islands are isolated in the South Pacific with one international seaport where natives had access to diets with industrialized nation's quantities of salt and native's blood pressures there were compared to subjects on an isolated island with natives consuming diets of fish and local vegetables with half the salt intake of the more modern island's population. The blood pressures of the sea port population steadily increased with age just as in developed countries, whereas the remote islands population's blood pressure remained stable as they aged.[4] Untreated 70-year-olds averaged pressures in the 120 mm range. Wow.

Reduction of salt to a nominal intake of just about a teaspoonful (3.5 grams) from over two teaspoons would reduce mortality in America from chronic disease by about 100,000 a year.[5] Just as many of the unhealthy behaviors small insults to the body are cumulative over decades.

Current CDC recommendations for people with hypertension, African Americans, and people over 40 years is less than 1.5 grams of sodium per day, which calculates as less than 3.5 grams of table salt. There is some confusion because sodium is consumed as salt (sodium chloride) so the weight changes by a factor of 2.5. A nickel weighs 5 grams. Nevertheless, the amount of salt in prepared foods you buy at the supermarket is often high. Read the nutritional labels and avoid overdosing on salt. Weigh yourself daily and you will observe that your weight will go up several pounds after consuming a high salt meal. The merchants will sell you food that will do you harm if you are not careful.

Such a widespread modest reduction in salt as recommended would be difficult to accomplish without altering the existing food supply. Read the nutritional labels, particularly the processed foods, especially the processed meats. Look at the nutritional labels for salt content and buy the least salted products.

Many years ago, medicine did not have the various medicines to treat hypertension it has now and salt reduction was a major treatment recommendation. Now, although unfortunate, fundamentals have become secondary to pharmacological advances.

With low-grade hypertension, modifications of lifestyle should be tried first, but if unsuccessful, medications should be started. There are a number of categories of medications available to treat hypertension. They are effective in different groups of patients and have different side effects. Those with mild to moderate hypertension should be started on single drug therapy that is effective in half of patients.

The single medications with the lowest side effects should be tried first using lower doses. The physician or pharmacist can inform about possible side effects. Combinations of antihypertensive medications can be used if a single medicine fails to meet therapeutic goals.

The take-home message of this chapter is that knowing about your health is important and participating in your hypertension treatment is essential.

Chapter 13

Happiness

What Is It? How Does One Grab It and Maximize It?

"The purpose of life is to be happy."

—Dalai Lama

WHAT REALLY IS HAPPINESS?

A number of things people consider important frequently are relegated to being just backdrops of life, including love and especially happiness. They will occur at the proper times because that is the way we are constructed. I recently had a good friend tell me, "I have never been a happy person. That is just the way I am." Well, each of us determines the way we are.

As Abraham Lincoln is said to have said, "Folks are usually about as happy as they make their minds up to be." Let's explore the questions, "What is really happiness? How does one grab it and maximize it?"

Ask anyone about happiness and they will agree that they know all they need to know. "I know it when I feel it," they say, but ask for a definition and they will stammer. And there will be many answers. This is because, like love, happiness cannot be willed, but the situation is comparable to becoming better financially by knowing financial wisdom; happiness is achievable by knowing how to harness it.

Happy is often used when we mean glad, pleased, joyful, or content. "Satisfied" is another word for which "happy" can be substituted. As in, "I'm happy the hailstorm didn't do more damage." Not really happiness.

Happiness is one of the greatest driving forces of human nature, barely behind self-preservation. It is right up there with unalienable rights of life and liberty in the Declaration of Independence. Actually, as we all know, we have a right to *pursue happiness* so it is important that we know how.

Happiness means many things to different people but that vagueness does not make it undefinable. Happiness is a mental status that is created from an emotion generated from living a good life. So, happiness is secondary to other things that we do to promote a "good life."

The "good life" concept goes back to the early Greek philosophers. The goal of life according to Plato's philosophy is to produce well-being and thus happiness. Plato considered the question, how best to attain the goal? The answer, he concluded, was, correct living produced well-being (i.e., living guided by the virtues). The virtues are ways of living, thus, the concept of cardinal virtues was created, ways of living to reach the "good life." They include: Fortitude (or Courage), Prudence, Temperance, and Justice.

Each of the virtues has a huge impact on promotion of the "good life" but the "golden mean" principle must be applied. Courage (standing up for your beliefs) must not be extreme. Too little of a stance is cowardice and when overdone courage becomes foolhardiness. Prudence allows self-governance because its closest synonym is forethought; prudence makes one decide beforehand, is this action likely beneficial or not? Applying prudence is being thoughtful and shunning impulsive actions.

Temperance is moderation in behavior. It says I will choose the correct amounts in my life. I read the other day a rich New Yorker tipped a server $500 and made the news. Other servers get shafted which is worse but the cultural tipping oil remains 15% to 20% of the tab according to the quality of service. Norms should be the norm. Justice is being messed with constantly now. Both twenty-three hundred years ago and today rational justice remains: give to him or to her what they truly contextually deserve—no less and no more.

"Fairness" has raised its ugly head, obscuring justice, in time fairness warps back over a century ago guessing what might have been if great-great-great-grandparents had acted differently, which is unreal. Justice applies to the here and now. A worker agrees or not to do specific tasks and gets paid as agreed, which is justice.

The famous German philosopher Georg Wilhelm Friedrich Hegel best defined true happiness as a reward you give yourself from attaining a desire. Most of our efforts are aimed at producing happiness when our goals are reached. We want to be liked, productive, and successful, and go to great lengths to achieve those goals. Pleasure in the way you are living is true earned happiness. I recently attended my 50th reunion from graduating Tulane Medical School and this year received the Outstanding Alumnus Award. Talk about happiness. Forgive me for tooting my own horn.

Three aspects of subjective well-being can be distinguished: evaluative wellbeing (or life satisfaction), hedonic well-being (transient feelings of happiness, pleasure), and eudemonic well-being (sense of purpose and meaning in life). In essence, the three represent evaluations of past, present, and future statuses.

We can find happiness where it resides, in the positive quality of our thoughts about people and events. Remember that every cloud, even rainclouds, have silver linings. Look for the silver linings. My grandmother Nichols was a nurse and was the happiest person I have ever known. I do not recall her ever saying anything bad about anyone, even real human rats, or being upset, even when my grandfather died unexpectedly in his early 60s. At his funeral she said, "He was a good man who meant well, even though he cursed like the sailor he was. He is in a much better place now." She died almost a half century later at 101 years, happy, alert, and loved by all. She told me once when I asked about life's hard knocks, "you just take what life gives you, hug it, and it will be alright."

The human being is the only animal that dotes on the future.[1] This observation is very important in determining whether to be happy or not. It introduces possibilities into the mix. The determination of happiness now is not based on whether I have all desired needs but, in addition, whether I will continue to have them. Uncertainty is cast into the mix. Uncertainty is unsettling by its very nature. My personal takeaway observation for the happiness bank is when I have considered the future, nothing I have thought would turn out bad turned out as bad as I considered it might be. And most everything I considered would be good, turned out to be better than I thought. Rational measured optimism is good for the soul.

THE VALUE OF HAPPINESS

Happiness is a strongly positive emotional mood, along with hope, inspiration, pride, gratitude, and love. I may have left some out but there aren't many more. Aside from happiness, the others are attached or directed to specifics, whereas happiness is an overall mental state that colors everything a shade better. Your worries about Aunt Nerm's health, finances, and even the dog

barking next door are not as troubling when the happiness factor is operative. Happiness is truly emotional rose colored glasses. It is the grease that
smooths out life.

Happiness levels are important factors in better and longer lives.[2]
The English Longitudinal Study of Aging examined the sense of purpose and
meaning in life (the "Good Life" of the Greeks) and found that those in the
lowest quartile died at three times the rate of those that were happiest in the
study interval. Happy Americans not only lived longer than unhappy ones,
but their longevity was increased according to the degree they experienced
happiness.[3] There is no question that positive emotions build or improve
physical health.[4]

In a large European study, the areas which provided the most meaning
were, as one might guess, family, work, and social relationships.[5] People who
felt those areas were alright were happier. We should make plans to improve
on any aspects of those areas we can and our persona will benefit or if all is
well, be grateful.

WHO IS HAPPIER?

There are a number of social measures where people are happier but I must
mention that the data is mostly from observational studies, which may show
causality but might not. For instance, older people that exercise are happier
but is exercise the reason or is the reason that healthier people are better able
to exercise? In a study where the data are more likely to show causality,
pedometers were used to measure the quantity of physical activity in older
adults and their measured physical activity correlated with their Satisfaction
with Life.[6] Want to be happier? *Start walking*.

There is some genetic influence on how happy an individual is: modestly
higher IQs were much happier than those below average.[7] The science here
may not be accurate because higher IQ may be a covariant with better lifestyle accruements. Regardless of how IQ attaches to happiness, it does so.
Get smarter. Be happier.

Money by itself does not promote happiness.[8] Lottery winners are not
happier even though they had huge windfalls.[9] In fact, within a short time
afterwards, they become unhappier as the result of being wealthy. Wealthy
people are presumed to be leading better lives but they have more tension and
spend fewer hours in leisure time. The lack of correlation between wealth and
happiness possibly is from the set point theory of happiness. As one accumulates more, expectations increase.

When I was in medical school, I had so little money that I could rarely afford lunch. I would slowly drink a 5-cent cup of coffee and get free refills while classmates at my table ate a full lunch; I was delighted when I could gobble a burger, usually at the beginning of the month just after payday. Now my happiness set-point has risen, so an expensive meal with wine is required now and it is the company that provides delights, not the food. Money does not beget happiness unless it provides a higher social status.[10]

Religion has a role in making people happier.[11] The happiness-enhancing effect of religion is strongest in countries where religion is most popular.[12] Religiosity has a protective effect in warding off depression by increasing resilience.[13] Religion seems a buffer against difficulties severe enough to restrict happiness. When disappointing events occur, it is human nature to have them echo in the mind. I had a Jewish friend and Jews are remarkably resilient; when disappointed, they would just shrug and say, "This too will pass."

WHAT NOT TO DO

Self-pity is generally referred to as a pity party. Those goings-on beat the crap out of happiness. When I was an intern at the esteemed Philadelphia General Hospital, now closed, one of the jobs was to collect blood from prisoners at the state prison. Prisoners would lie down on cots on a basketball court to donate blood and receive $5. Loud be-bop-a-lula music played in the background. I would go from one cot to another inserting needles and assistants would collect the blood. One day the guards had machine guns rather than clubs. I asked, "What is going on?" "These are the worst of the worst," a guard replied. "They will only go out of here in a box."

I passed down the aisle inserting needles and, yes, I was glad they were locked up. Then I approached an inmate with a big "Howdy Doody" smile. "You seem extraordinarily happy," I said. "Doc, here I am lying flat on my back in the middle of the day, listenin' to good music, and makin' five dollars. I got it made." For almost a half century, when I feel a pity party coming on, I remember that moment and think or shout, if I am alone, "Hell, I got it made" and everything straightens out.

Criticism poisons happiness unless viewed as valuable and therefore positive. It depends on how it is presented. It is best given as questioning the wisdom of actions as in: "Do you think another action would have been better?" Avoid proclaiming: "You really screwed up" even if true. People enjoy being correct; they don't enjoy being wrong. Perhaps, that is the reason why educational level is important in determining the happiness level.

Presently there is a constant barrage of unpleasant information, part of which is news. One should limit exposure to unpleasant news. I hardly watch or listen to the news anymore because it is easy to overdose. News reporters, especially those on the news channels, collect everything bad that has recently happened. News rarely reports the millions of good self-sacrificing events because humans are fascinated by tragedy much more than everyday good deeds. Otherwise, rubbernecking would not be a universal practice on highways.

It is true evil that seems to flourish in the twenty-first century with unspeakable horror from the Middle East to classrooms in America. We must consider all events both good and bad in perspective. Within the lifetime of most of you reading this, the Second World War resulted in hundreds of times more deaths than all that has transpired since 9/11.[14]

Regret is an emotion where we face the fact we could have acted differently and avoided an unfortunate outcome. It is reliving a bad time with guilt superimposed. It is traveling through life looking through a rear view mirror—not wise. We need to learn from our mistakes and then travel onward without suffering guilt by revisiting the situation with regret. If one learns from his or her past, the past is closed as a meaningful experience and does not need to be relived.

WHERE IS HAPPINESS TO BE FOUND?

One of the principal venues for happiness is to look where there is meaning. Meaning according to a modern philosopher Robert Nozick requires communication with other intelligent beings. As mentioned, but worth repeating, the most valuable painting in the world according to Guinness World Records is the *Mona Lisa*. It is insured for over a half billion dollars. It has a great deal of meaning in addition to its value but if it were preserved in a locked vault where no one could appreciate it, it would retain value but lose meaning.

Previously, I was intrigued and reported information from Dr. Eagleman's book *Incognito: Secret Lives of the Brain*, where his thesis was our brains work almost autonomously without our awareness. Our subconscious brains are continuously processing information and answers bubble to the surface as our consciousness proclaims, "Aha!" An excellent metaphor, from another author Dr. Haidt, is that our consciousness is similar to the rider of an elephant; the rider has limited control because the elephant can go anywhere it wishes. When observing a cute baby or pet, don't you smile and suddenly feel better? Contrarily, have you ever just met someone who you immediately disliked only to realize they reminded you of a past offender? Smiling or frowning tells the elephant how it should behave. Women given Botox injections to reduce wrinkles from frowning are happier.[15]

So, smile more and frown less.

Part III

MEDICAL CARE AND MANAGEMENT

Chapter 14

Understanding the Basics of How Medical Care Works

IMPORTANCE OF UNDERSTANDING THE FUNDAMENTALS OF MEDICINE

Understanding the fundamentals of medical practice is a tremendous advantage for laypeople because they and their loved ones will require future medical care. Medical therapy works better when divested of mysticism and when it is a participatory effort.

Patients cannot effectively participate in decisions about their healthcare without understanding the process. Understanding healthcare improves the chance they will make the best decisions about when to seek care, who should provide that care, and what care to agree to have.

I always tried to tell patients undergoing major surgery what to expect and I am convinced they had a smoother postoperative course. "You will be surrounded by a group of masked professionals who will have for the next few hours a total dedication to making you well. What seems like an instant later, you will awaken in your hospital room with monitors and strange noises to assure those taking care of you that you are doing well. If at any time, there is a problem, you will be immediately told. So, relax and be assured; everything is as it should be. You are on your way to beating this problem."

The unknown when concerning your health, and especially your life, can be terrifying. Anxiety causes release of hormones and other stressors that prepare the body for action against a threat. These factors are unhealthy, promoting or worsening chronic disease. Life is a marathon, not a sprint. All medical situations courses should be clarified to reduce anxiety. If no explanation is forthcoming, ask "Doctor, what should I expect will happen in the course of my treatment?"

To secure quality medical care, just as in securing health, patients must fulfill their responsibilities and, first, they must know about their responsibilities. Patients must seek medical care as early as possible when care is needed. Trying to determine when care is needed is not difficult. There are certain symptoms which should get your attention and we will go over those in a later chapter about red flags. Doctors have support personnel, nurses, and others who can give advice about what to do. Patients need to interact with a basic common sense participation in their care and be compliant with recommendations or tell the doctor why they don't follow prescribed therapy. The main reason I wrote this book is that after retirement I became a patient and realized the advantages basic information about health and medical care could give. I have doctors and made a pact that I will do whatever I am instructed to do after rational consideration or find another doctor. That is excellent advice for everyone.

First, I will try to give a brief statement about the nature of physicians, and then briefly describe the marvelous complexity of the body we inhabit. It will amaze that disorders don't occur more frequently. Then we will examine practical medical practice through generalities.

PHYSICIANS AND OTHER CAREGIVERS ARE HUMAN

First, and most obvious, physicians are well-trained humans with all the associated frailties. Patients tend to forget that at times because it is a lot more reassuring to put your life in the hands of a superlative person. We bestow exalted status on those performing important tasks for us. My minister is a special person because he has the ability to reassure in difficult times and one supposes he has extraordinary connections with God. However, my reliance on suggestions he makes requires rational examination, as should be the case when receiving medical therapy.

Once, early in my career, when I was working in an emergency room, I examined a youngster who had an obvious case of appendicitis. When I told the parents that the child must have his appendix removed, they insisted I call their family physician. He was not available for hours, dangerous hours, but regardless the parents would not give consent. Had refusal continued, I would have awakened a judge. When and only when their physician, who was not a surgeon, agreed, did they allow the operation to proceed. Fortunately, the child recovered.

Trust should always be rational relative to realism. I employed a lawn-man and was pleased for years, but then some of his newly hired employees began to mow hurriedly, leaving gaps. When I spoke to the yardman, he explained my yard, and not his employee's mowing, was at fault. I hired a new lawn-man. If someone employed by you, including physicians, gives you explanations that don't make sense, find someone else. The overwhelming number of physicians nowadays explain things very well. Medicine is not rocket science; we just use big Latin words. Medicine's difficulty rests in the volume of knowledge, not its complexity. This may change as we begin to explore gene and immunotherapy.

To be most effective, physicians need to remain objective by remaining emotionally detached. Liking someone too much can alter perceptions so that subjectivity skews actions. Most physicians do not treat relatives or close friends for fear they cannot perform objectively which is necessary to execute optimally. In the past, it was considered that physicians received poorer medical care than the general public because it was tempting for another doctor to do something special for them, euphemistically termed a "blue plate special." The American Medical Association (AMA) cautions physicians about treating patients close to them. Highly competent physicians establish their own clinical processes over years and thousands of patient encounters and must guard against deviations except for the direst circumstances.

Many physicians, especially older surgeons, have superstitions because of past experiences. A common belief is that bad clinical outcomes happen in pairs or threes. It seemed to me that whenever a patient or their family gave me something, even a thank you card, while still hospitalized, their care became more complicated. Silly? Perhaps.

Don't assume your physician has special powers. Don't even assume they have your past medical history completely in mind. If your symptoms seem to be getting worse, it is time to visit your physician and make sure they know your medical history. Keep a record of your medical care. Include dates of medicine changes, lab results, and procedures. Microsoft Excel works well for that purpose.

Doctors are under continuing pressure to be more efficient, which translates to spending less time with each patient. Except for boutique medicine, the leisurely thoroughness of the past is disappearing fast. And ever-increasing reams of government regulations and health insurance hoops are unavoidable distractions.

Your doctor knows the generalities of your disease but you know the specifics. Keep a log when your condition seems to change. My personal physician is recognized as being at the top of his specialty. He prescribed a new medication and I developed annoying tingling. He had never had a patient develop tingling from that medication and did not think the medication caused it. I stopped the medicine and the tingling stopped. He then, when I notified him, had a patient who had tingling from that medicine.

HOW TO CHOOSE YOUR PHYSICIAN

All docs are not created equal. There was an old joke in medical school that went like this: "What do you call the student that graduates last in his class?" Doctor is the answer. Medical schools don't graduate incapable doctors but there is a difference in quality. After medical school, additional training is required. There is a vaunted medical honor society, the AOA (Alpha Omega Alpha Honor Medical Society). It is the Phi Beta Kappa of medical school. Doctors having that designation's grades were in the top few and they were elected by members of the society, which is a good start.

I want a smart doctor because medicine requires good decision making from good judgment. Experience is the additional factor which contributes to medical decision making. A famous surgeon that was a friend used to pontificate about medical practice, "Good judgement comes from experience and experience comes from bad judgement." A quote from Will Rogers but then he would grin and add, "But the bad judgement doesn't have to be yours."

A primary care doctor is the manager of your medical care. The kind of doctor you need and kind in medicine means the specialty of doctor which depends on several factors. Several specialists that provide primary care for adults include: family practitioners, OB/GYN, general internal medicine, and gerontologists.

Family practitioners provide primary care for all ages. OB/GYN docs provide primary care for women. The general internal medicine docs specialize in diseases of the internal organs including the heart and lungs which is what older people need to have evaluated, which makes them well suited for those who are aging. Gerontologists specialize in overall care of the aging body and are recommended for those who have complicated diseases of the elderly.

Being asked to join a sizable medical group practice is a good sign. Having board certification in the specialty of practice is minimal. Renowned medical institutions have high standards for their doctors especially procedure performers. It always amazed me that the overriding criterion for many patients is convenience in choosing medical care. Some will drive further to a good restaurant than to seek quality medical care. Routine uncomplicated care can be taken care of almost anywhere but when undergoing complex procedures seek the best you can find. The more complicated the care needed, the more care you should take in finding a caregiver.

Another way people choose physicians is from their friends' recommendations. What makes them think their friends have any expertise about the quality of their medical care? Most judge a doc on the basis of whether they like them, which is the wrong criterion. Many docs that are busy because they are capable may seem rushed or even curt when just the opposite is true. It is an added benefit to connect with the doc but don't choose because you are liking the doc; you are not going to a medical clinic to have another friend.

I was with a world class surgeon who was visiting a dignitary before an operation and was asked by the dignitary whether he was going to listen to the patient's heart. The noted surgeon said, "no, I don't listen to hearts, I fix hearts," then he turned about and walked out of the room. Your doc should listen to you concerning your ailments but don't confuse or substitute attentiveness with competence.

One older, very smart friend esteems his physician because the doc gives out medicine samples. Really? Drug samples exist to promote the more expensive drugs, not the less expensive generics. I did not inform him of the fact that he was likely paying more than needed but my mouth was agape. A little knowledge goes a long way in noting what is actually going on in your medical care.

There is a way to find out where doctors of a particular specialty would go or take their families for specialty medical care: "Best Doctors in America." There are other so-called best doctors but many of their doctors pay to be included. Recommended doctors from "Best Doctors in America" are elected by others in the same specialty in their region. The Best Doctors in America's question is simple: "Would you go to this doctor if you needed treatment provided in your medical specialty?" There is no charge for inclusion. As a member for years, I remember that the most respected of my specialty were on the ballot and those included only represented the top few. The real "Best Doctors" has a blue square with white dots composing a cross and a star near the center. Their website address is bestdoctors.com.

American medicine overall is the best in the world but you should only settle for the best of the best, especially when you need procedures. It will benefit you in the end.

Search for a physician who questions you in detail and examines you in a thoughtful manner. If you have a complaint about a certain area of your body, your physician should examine it—look, touch, and if necessary listen to it. Too many physicians order unnecessary tests to make the diagnosis[1] which is costly and may be misleading. Overutilization of medical care is about three times as frequent as underutilization.[2] Second opinions are much more common than in the past and can be reassuring.

WHEN AND HOW TO PARTICIPATE IN YOUR CARE

Patients should resolutely participate in their care by interacting at key junctures. Key junctures are identified by changes in therapy or when new symptoms arise. When a new medication is being prescribed, patients should ask whether it will interact with what they are taking, to be certain their doctor reviews their medication list. The physician should be able to avoid problems by not prescribing drugs that interact. There are a huge number of subtle less severe interactions that may be found easily on the web. Two of the best drug interaction checkers are at AARP and Medscape; both are excellent. Ask and then check the websites.

Ask about common side effects with a "what should I be on the lookout for in untoward effects" question. Pharmacies give out information with prescriptions and it should be read, but the list is fashioned to protect the pharmaceutical companies legally and is incredibly long. So, ask your doctor, as they write the prescription, what you should look out for. They will have seen the common side effects and should be aware of the dangerous ones.

Certainly with any significant change in therapy, one should inquire about details, especially how to go about achieving the goals and how to know when the goals have been achieved. For instance, if told to get more exercise, ask about specifics. If the medical treatment is complex write down or record the instructions. Carry a notepad and pencil to appointments.

Some patients hesitate to question their physicians because they fear they may cause offense. Your doctor wants to provide you with the best care possible and having an actively participating patient is desirable. Not just in medicine, wanting to know more about a service usually encourages the provider to a higher level. In the past, some physicians were paternal in demeanor but that has diminished with the rise in patient autonomy. We used to simply tell patients what was to be done and they accepted it. Now, the patients need to understand what is to be done to their bodies and why and agree to accept the recommendation.

Before office visits, a little preparation will be beneficial. Aside from general checkups, note the main reason for the appointment, in medical terminology that is your "chief complaint." Most often, the chief complaint is simple, like "I fell on the steps and twisted my ankle." However, in more vague situations, describe your chief complaint in detail. How long has it been going on? Have you experienced it before? Bring a list of the questions you want answered so they won't be overlooked.

Most of us want to get the most value for a visit. It is alright to bring an agenda with a number of things for consideration. Deal completely with the chief complaint first to avoid distracting the doctor. When finished with the treatment phase of your chief complaint, it is the proper time to discuss other matters – one at a time.

The determination that an illness is caused by a specific disease becomes a patient's diagnosis. Initially, the diagnostic process is set in motion by a patient's description of their illness. In medical terms this becomes that patient's "chief complaint" and a more complete description is the "present illness." In many office visits, especially to a primary care provider, the illness is a common one such as a cold or a sprain needing little detective work. In these straightforward cases, the diagnosis is obvious because it may be influenza season or as mentioned the patient tells of twisting their ankle. If it quacks and looks like a duck, it probably is a duck. An old pearl was "if you hear hoof-beats, don't think of a zebra." In other words, look for the common diseases first.

The other method of diagnosing is more involved and is termed "differential diagnosis" when two or more diseases that could cause the same illness are considered. Chest pain has many causes and through the history one can list the several most likely diseases. It would be important to determine the character of the pain. Is it sharp or dull? Is it continuous or intermittent? Does it start somewhere and radiate elsewhere? What activities bring it on? Make it worse? What relieves it? These descriptors should be noted in describing all types of pain leading to a medical visit.

The physical exam consists of the physician first observing the area where the problem is thought to arise. Next, the exam proceeds to touching the area (palpating) and/or listening (auscultation) with a stethoscope. If the area has tender muscles, the problem is likely musculoskeletal. If a rib is tender, it is possibly a fracture or inflammation. Laboratory tests and X-rays allow the elimination of specific diagnoses to arrive at the most likely one which is then treated.

In certain instances, especially in emergency situations, when the diagnosis is yet to be determined but one or more of the possibilities is serious, the therapy is directed toward the more serious diagnosis and the diagnosis is termed a "working diagnosis." In the case of a patient with chest pain seen in the ER, it is prudent to assume it comes from the heart and the patient is treated as if they have heart trouble as they are tested until it is determined not to be the case.

Patients can assist in their initial diagnosis by preparing a description of their illness and writing it down. There is an old medical tale about a farmer who developed tetanus and went to the doctor with a sore throat. The doc looked at Sam's throat and said there was nothing wrong and he should gargle with salt water. Sam came back each day complaining of worsening sore throat. On the third day, Sam said, "Doc, my throat is so sore I can't swallow anything. Do you think it could be lockjaw from that pitchfork I stepped on?" Yup.

Cost of medical care is important but rarely is considered. Cost should not be the determining factor for therapy but merits consideration just as side effects of the therapy.[3] A discussion of what a patient's out-of-pocket expenses are likely to be is important in expensive treatments. Some treatments have astronomical price tags and seeking early financial aid may be warranted. If the medical bills are accumulating or generating a problem, the patient needs to talk to the business manager to make arrangements.

THERAPY IN A NUTSHELL

After the diagnosis is made, the course of a disease (its natural history) becomes important to decide therapy or no therapy. The usual course of different diseases has been studied over time, usually before there was an adequate treatment for a particular disease. Natural history focuses on what will happen over time if the disease is not treated. Using this knowledge the doctor stages the disease as to whether it is early or advanced. In general more advanced disease states are more difficult to treat and have more complications. This is especially important in potentially terminal diseases such as cancer.

When a major procedure is recommended, patients have the right to have informed consent before deciding whether or not to have it performed.

Informed consent has several parts. What would happen without the procedure, all possible treatments, why a particular treatment is recommended, what is the expectation of success, and what are the complications related to the procedure. All of the information necessary for the patient to make a decision should be disclosed.

An important fact to be determined, especially if the procedure is relatively new, is: How many and how often does the doctor do this procedure? The "learning curve," especially concerning newly minted procedures is important. Procedures that have "learning curves" have more chances of things going wrong until a sufficient experience is gained. Also, in teaching hospitals, you want to know how much of the procedure is to be done by a supervised resident in training. Usually, in teaching hospitals where residents are being supervised, the care is excellent because the supervising doctor is fully trained and his/her reputation is at stake.

The worse the possible outcome of a disease (prognosis), the more daringly medicine deals with it. No one would consider radical surgery for minor skin conditions. Radical excision of a potentially lethal cancer is understandable.

Doctors treat diseases by noting what is malfunctioning and counteracting the excess or replacing the deficiencies. When the thyroid produces too much thyroid hormone, initially the treatment was to remove part of the gland. Later, a radioisotope was injected that killed the overproductive thyroid cells intentionally causing deficiency of thyroid hormone that is replaced in normal amounts.

Almost all therapies have associated problematic results. Surgical procedures harm before they heal. Some of the complications are quite serious. Coronary bypass procedures in small percentages of patients results in a stroke or even a heart attack during the procedure. The surgeon examines likely outcomes of alternatives to surgery including doing nothing against the risk factors of each patient that gives an idea of the outcome of an operation. If the benefits clearly outweigh the risks, the procedure is indicated. If not, the procedure is contraindicated. In all patients there will be pain and some disability during the recovery period. To reduce the postoperative pain and the recovery time, an entirely new series of operative procedures have been developed, the minimally invasive procedures, which use several small incisions rather than one large one.

There is a hierarchy in medicine especially with complex surgical procedures. There is a difference between knowing something and knowing how to do something. Medical school teaches knowing something, whereas the how-to-do is experiential. Both are important but in surgery and almost all procedures, the how to do is the most important. There is clearly a "learn-ing curve" in performing procedures; it is seen in every scientific article that examines results in new procedures. The learning curve is why years are required in residency under supervision by experienced surgeons. Even fully trained surgeons need to keep a certain level of experience to produce optimal outcomes.

SELECTING A SURGEON

There are three reasons why to select a surgeon who is busy doing the proce-dure you need. They likely are better at it than someone doing it less often. Many of the good and especially the great technical surgeons operate on automatic pilot. That is they can talk to their assistants as though they were in the doctor's lounge and do complex technical maneuvers. One famous surgeon stated, "The best surgeon's motor impulses never reach their cortex." Meaning they have done that so many times they don't have to think; it's automatic. It's not a derogatory concept. Did Babe Ruth have to think, "Now, that's a hittable ball, I will swing at that pitch."

And when a surgeon encounters a bend in the road, if experienced, they automatically go into a subroutine. When you first learned to tie your shoes, it was awkward but with experience became automatic. The more skilled a surgeon is, the less wasted motion there is and the operation is done better and faster.

Second, surgery, except perhaps cosmetic surgery, depends on referrals. Unless the different docs are in the same clinic, referring docs refer patients to surgeons who get the best results. The surgeon who is the busiest has the most referring docs who are the most satisfied with his or her work.

Last, the busiest surgeon's work is likely to cost you less. A real busy surgeon cannot remain busy when many patients have complications. Com-plications take a lot of time and effort to heal. Complications are expensive; they can easily triple the hospital bill. And even those with insurance, have copays that are substantial.

Several years back, I needed a procedure that differed from my specialty. I contacted two internationally known surgeons who I had helped teach them how to do heart surgery with a single question, "Who at your institution does the most of this procedure?" I made an appointment with their suggested cardiologist and did well. The number of procedures always trumps. This is especially important when the procedure is new. Procedures, especially those requiring new skill sets, have a learning curve. Newer is not always better; remember the Affordable Care Act website's problems.

Not just surgery has undesirable side effects, medications especially those that alter general bodily functions have long lists of untoward effects. One has only to read their medication's printed inserts to see the wide range of untoward effects that can result from using a drug. Patient's allergic reactions to medicines are a good example and can be quite serious. Doctors therefore must develop good judgment because medical practice is often as much an art as it is a science.

Some therapies take time to resolve illnesses. It is useful to know what one should expect from a treatment. A simple "when should I start to feel better" will provide the answer.

Chapter 15

Red Flags

Early Alerts for Age-Lifestyle-Related Diseases

Age-lifestyle-related diseases are the deadliest threats to health in America, which is why death rates increase as we age. Seventy percent of all American deaths and 92% of deaths in people over 65 years are from those diseases. Age-related disease's cures are directly related to how advanced they are when treatment begins, which should emphasize the importance of this chapter on early recognition. Those who do not know what a rattlesnake's rattle sounds like are more likely to get snake-bit in the wilderness. A rattle is a red flag warning that defensive action is necessary to avoid serious problems; knowing the red flags your body flies permit prompt treatment that is more effective. Earlier treatment is always more successful because time allows the disease to damage tissues and worsen. Damage that destroys tissue structure may not be repaired because treatment stops the damage; repair is up to the body.

I do not want to alarm anyone excessively. I do strongly believe that in important matters of heath and disease, if one errs, one should err on the side of caution. What I am classifying as "red flags" are warning signs that conceivably indicate manifestations of treatable diseases. It is wise to investigate red flags. My car recently developed a new noise coming from the engine compartment. I immediately made a service department appointment to be sure that further damage did not accrue. A repair was made that left unattended would have been much more expensive. Our health is certainly more important than our cars.

A guiding principle in medicine is the risk/benefit ratio; it considers possible costs of a certain action versus the possible benefits the action could

151

provide. Costs of becoming overly concerned about an inconsequential finding are an unnecessary doctor's appointment. Benefits of early detection of health problems are incalculable.

I class changes in our bodies or behavior in terms of the three categories in the title of the old Clint Eastwood movie: *The Good, the Bad, and The Ugly*. First, the good: I am adopting some of the behavioral suggestions in a book by Dr. Amit Sood entitled *The Mayo Clinic Gide to Stress-Free Living*. My life is better even if my changes only are because I believe they are better. Growing (becoming more skilled in living well) was emphasized as we were growing up but we should never stop growing. Old dogs can make changes in lifestyles that are more beneficial than when they were young dogs because they have more to lose because they have less reserve than young dogs. Reserve preservation is important as life lengthens.

Bad red flags are on what we will focus because they are the majority of red flags that if treated early have better outcomes. Almost any red flag, as recognized, must be dealt with as a potential threat; most will be from easy-to-remedy changes or treatments or will allow successful early treatment solutions. The ugly red flags are the harbingers announcing the few conditions for which medicine has no good solution. Fortunately, they are a distinct minority and are continually decreasing as medical knowledge progresses.

GENERAL FACTORS

Note your overall well-being daily. What is your energy level? Are you feeling more tired lately? Are you requiring more sleep? We all have intermingled good days and bad days but when a pattern of decreasing energy becomes obvious, it indicates a major change in our body. The possibilities range from easily correctable, such as thyroid medication, or finding and correcting matters that are more serious.

One notable cause of decreasing energy as we age is sleep apnea (pauses in breathing during sleep). This is often common among men who snore and who do not breathe for periods followed by gasping. A spouse can provide the diagnostic information. It can be corrected with a breathing machine or a dental prosthesis if mild. Having sleep apnea treated will provide double benefit both to you and your spouse.

Decreasing energy can also be due to anemia. As we age the chance of becoming iron deficient increases because blood loss may be unappreciated. Anemia is surprisingly common in the elderly; it occurs at a rate of 20% in elderly men and 13% in women.[1] Take a look at the redness of your palms in comparison to your special other's palms periodically and if it noticeably changes get checked. In men and post-menopausal women anemia is likely an early sign of GI bleeding, which needs investigation.

Our energy is dampened if some of our glands stop secreting the amounts of hormones we need. In particular, the thyroid has inadequate secretions in both women and men (more common in women). Signs and symptoms include: fatigue, sensitivity to cold, difficulty sleeping, depression, and bowel changes, mainly constipation. When overall energy decreases hormone levels should be measured.

Sudden changes in behavior in adults are often ugly red flags. A common cause of behavioral changes is medications, especially new meds. Emotional outbursts, forgetfulness of commonly traveled routes, withdrawal from close contacts, decreased ability to function, and especially these defects when noticed by others can signal the onset of diseases, both mental and physical, which need attention.

Everyone should weigh themselves regularly. Unintended changes in weight are real red flags. Gains and especially unintended losses of over 5% within several months should result in a doctor visit. I had an older friend who belonged to the same coffee group and I noticed he was losing weight. He told me that he had lost 20 pounds in the last few months. My response was to encourage him to see a diagnostician I recommended. A week later, he stated that he would visit relatives in two weeks and would schedule an appointment afterwards. He died during the visit to his relatives of an easily treatable stomach condition.

WHAT TO DO ABOUT RED FLAGS

There is a distinct advantage to promptly dealing with red flags. The answer to better health is mainly preventative but prevention has its limits and early detection of problems is a good second line of defense. Over half of elderly (over 65 years) have had at least one chronic disease diagnosed and when a diagnosis can be made it represents advanced disease.

I frequently hear people say that they are disappointed in the length of time it takes to get an appointment with a specialist when they are concerned about a red flag. First, a busy doc is a respectable sign of good medical practice. Long delays can feed discomfort and worry, especially if you are in pain. The scheduling person is usually not medically trained and you might ask if the appointment can be moved up. State that you would be willing to wait in the office until you could be fitted in or that you would be willing to come in if there was a cancellation. If that doesn't work, call your primary care doc's office. They have a great deal more clout with specialists because they are their source of referral. Use your primary care doc's influence; they and their office staff are usually more than happy to be helpful—if not change docs.

Chronic physical disease in the elderly frequently appears early as behavioral changes. Mild cognitive decline associated with noticeable depression, anxiety, or irritability should be investigated. Recurring sudden feelings of hopelessness (dysphoria) are notable red flags.

SPECIFICS, ESPECIALLY PAIN

Pain is the most common beacon of protection we have. Pain notifies us we have an injury or are being injured and makes us withdraw and rest the injured part until it has recovered. Pain is unpleasant and teaches us to avoid behaviors that could be harmful. Pain is mental as well as physical. Mental pain is more complex than physical pain and since my qualifications are limited with mental pain and it is less deadly, we shall concentrate on physical pain.

Going to see a doctor for pain is so obvious; you probably wonder why I would mention it. Well, there are several types of pain, which are regularly misunderstood as innocent when they are not. A good example is back pain located in the flanks is likely not spinal; it can be from kidney disease and needs to be checked. Likewise, upper abdominal pain that radiates to the back often is an abdominal problem, not a back problem. Newly onset back pain (or any pain) that continues for over a week should be evaluated.

There are different types of pain and the character can lead the doctor to suspect certain causes. Aching pain is often muscular or skeletal in origin. It is most often steady and worsens with movement. The diagnosis is confirmed if the pain is reproduced by pressure on the area where the pain is located. In general, musculoskeletal pain can be troublesome but is among the least dangerous pains. It is most often from an injury or arthritis, recognized or not, not an underlying more dangerous pathology.

However, the deadliest warning pain we can have is from the heart and it is frequently masked. Heart pain heralding serious heart disease is angina. Everyone knows angina is serious. What they don't know is that in a substantial number of people angina is atypical; it may appear as indigestion or jaw pain. One patient I performed a quadruple bypass operation on had thousands of dollars of dental work done before his heart disease was diagnosed.

Insufficient blood flow to the heart from artery obstructions occurs when the heart has to work harder. This reduction in flow with exertion begins when the cross-sectional area of an artery is reduced by 70%. Symptoms result when the heart works harder and the demand can be from either physical or emotional exertion. Imagine what would happen when several lanes become closed on a major expressway; traffic blockages would be different at rush hour or three o'clock in the morning. Angina should be suspected when severe chest, abdominal, or jaw pain occurs with exertion and goes away when exertion ceases.

Angina does not mean pain, although it is commonly used as though it does. It comes from a Greek root meaning "to strangle." The same root gives us the words "anxiety" and "anguish," which angina certainly causes. The most common description is a feeling of pressure and not being able to breathe. Most commonly, patients say, "It feels like an elephant is standing on my chest." Be very concerned with any pain located on the left side of the chest that lasts over a minute. This is especially worrisome if the pain goes into your left arm. Chest pain that lasts for less than a minute is probably not angina but should be investigated.

About one-third of men have "silent ischemia" so they do not have angina to warn them to back off of what they are doing.[2] Angina warns that blockages of the heart's arteries are restricting blood flow and should be investigated. A stress test will validate that blockages are present or that the pain is not from the heart. An angiogram will determine the danger of the blockages and the treatment indicated.

The diseased area then can have a clot form and close the artery completely; heart attacks usually occur from clots and are termed "coronary thrombosis." Heart attacks occur rapidly (be concerned about any undesirable symptom that occurs rapidly) and fully get your attention, even if you have not had angina to warn you. Most people having a heart attack have an overwhelming sense of dread. They feel like a goner. Also, consider discomfort accompanied by sweating when you are not hot and or nausea to be serious.

Pain from skin is precisely located and of a specific character but pain from our internal organs is different. It is conveyed from the autonomic nervous system, which more properly could be called the automatic nervous system. It allows all sorts of things to happen without us thinking about them: breathing, digestion, heartbeat, and many more. The autonomic nervous system has two parts: the sympathetic and the parasympathetic. The sympathetic relays pain and sweating, ergo, heart pain has sweating.

Another possible clot-related pain is tenderness in a calf associated with ankle swelling. Ankle swelling in itself signals problems with circulation that need clarification by means of a diagnosis. However, sudden swelling that has not been there before, especially associated with a sore calf, indicates a possible blood clot. Such clots in the leg have a tendency to dislodge and go to the lungs—called a pulmonary embolus. Pulmonary emboli are a major cause of sudden death.

Back pain that radiates into the buttocks or legs, especially if associated with numbness, can be a herniated disc. Radiating pain into legs or arms is pain from nerve irritation, usually from compression.

Cramping pain is what most of us have experienced as gas pains, which occurs in hollow muscular organs (HMOs) when distended. Our HMOs are varied and plentiful. The GI tract has the most with the esophagus, stomach, liver and pancreas ducts, small bowel, large bowel, and rectum. The genito-urinary system is a close second with the ureters, bladder, urethra, and uterus. All the HMOs are sensitive to vigorous contractions and the distention it causes. Cramps can be initiated by blockages, which reflexly result in more vigorous contractions as the organ tries to empty. The blockages can be from stone formations as with kidney stones or gallstones or the bowel can become twisted. Some cramps are part of life such as menstrual cramps and gas pain but one should have new severe or persistent cramps investigated.

Headaches are another common source of pain. Sudden onset of the worst headache ever should prompt a call to 911. It could signal a weakened artery that is about to rupture. Also, one should become concerned when new recurring headaches begin in older adults, especially if severe enough to suspend daily activities. Headaches that are brought on with exertion or emotional stress should be investigated. Headaches that are located on one side of the head rather than general are worrisome. Headaches have many causes and most are of little consequence: Inconsequential headaches are infrequent and are similar to what was experienced in the past.

RED FLAGS BY ORGANS

Brain

Going into a room and forgetting why you went there is part of aging. Going into a room and not knowing where you are is a real red flag. Being unable to grasp the right word and later remembering it is annoying but all right. Stopping in the middle of a conversation and being unable to continue is a red flag. It is normal to become irritated when a regular routine is interrupted; it is abnormal to have wide fluctuations in mood (confusion, anger, suspicious, anxious, or fearful) without reason. Stating that mental functioning that seriously interferes with daily living summarizes dementia's danger signals is a real red flag.

OTHER RED FLAGS INDICATING VASCULAR DISEASE

Strokes are often preceded by heralding symptoms. These transient symptoms are termed "TIAs" (transient ischemic attacks) and just as the phrase implies, there is an abrupt functional difficulty that goes away with time. One may notice sudden difficulty speaking or weakness of a hand or leg which goes away usually within hours. One may just be confused, and this is more than a forgetful word "episode," about a matter. Sudden confusion such as losing track of conversation warrants investigation. When the problem goes away without medical care, an abrupt functional difficulty should never be dismissed as "just growing older." These sudden disturbing episodes are small clots lodging in the minute arteries of one's brain which temporarily cause a malfunction that goes away when the clot dissolves. Don't consider that because it resolves, it isn't dangerous. It will recur and likely will involve larger clots, which can kill cells in the brain causing a stroke. Before brain cells die and a stroke occurs, the problem can be corrected medically.

Skin

Skin warts and especially moles can become cancerous, as well as new lesions that seem to sprout up. Skin cancers are more common on areas exposed to the sun including the face and neck. Those people who have had a lot of exposure to sun should have new or changes in blemishes examined by a dermatologist. Changes in the size or color, especially of dark moles should arouse suspicion. If a lesion starts to develop an open sore, persistently itches, or bleeds without injury, a dermatologist should be consulted.

GASTROINTESTINAL RED FLAGS

Changes in bowel habits can be red flags. Diarrhea that starts suddenly and is associated with pain is a red flag. Jaundice is a red, red flag. It means bile salts are building up in one's body, causing it to turn yellow. The best place to look for jaundice's yellowing is in the whites of the eyes and the best examination is done in sunlight rather than artificial indoor light. Yellowing of the skin is preceded usually by light colored stool and dark urine. When dark urine is corrected by increasing water intake, it usually means one is dehydrated. Dehydration is not a dangerous red flag specifically but chronic dehydration predisposes to blood clots, which can be dangerous. Armpits should be slightly moist and the skin of the forearm should snap back promptly when pinched.

Bleeding gets attention; or does it? Bleeding that is unnoticed is most often from the gastrointestinal tract. The reason it may be unnoticed is that exposure to stomach acid or intestinal enzymes alters blood's color and texture. Vomitus containing blood has the appearance of coffee grounds. It may or may not have partly digested food or brownish green intestinal juices depending on when consumption of food occurred but stuff looking like coffee grounds means partially digested blood is also present. Digested blood that exists from the other end of the GI tract appears like sticky black tar. These are termed "tarry stools." Occasionally, when eating certain foods such as a rare steak, stools will be blackened. If one takes iron tablets, the stools will darken.

Our bodies are equipped with alarm systems and it is essential we recognize when the alarm goes off.

Chapter 16

Practical Medication Information
Improving Your Personal Medical Care

THE IMPORTANCE OF KNOWING ABOUT MEDICATIONS

There are often many ways to do things, even taking your meds. But there is always a best way and a little knowledge about your medicines can be of considerable benefit in discovering the best way. I have always believed, as Gertrude Stein, the noted author, quipped, "to be a difference, it has to make a difference." So, what follows either is proven to make a difference, or common sense from available facts make a difference very likely.

"Unfortunately, there's a disconnect between what's taught to doctors and what we know from chronotherapy research [when to take meds]," says circadian biologist Georgios Paschos of the University of Pennsylvania School of Medicine.[1] "Except for a few conditions, clinical medicine hasn't yet caught up with our findings." Nevertheless, he predicts, this will change in the next decade or two. I propose to catch you up right now in this chapter concerning the best way to organize your medical treatments.

What Dr. Paschos laments is that research investigating how to provide better medical results by timing medications is known but has not found its way into clinical medical practice. Delayed clinical application is not a new drawback; medicine broadly divides into two camps: physicians (MDs) who concentrate on providing and researching patient care and "basic scientists" (mainly PhDs) who concentrate on researching how our bodies work, how disease disrupts the workings, and how medicine works to correct disease.

159

Having both degrees (MD and PhD) and experience in both disciplines, I appreciate how both work and that their professional communications are primarily group-based. A while back, an attempt to bridge the information gap foraged for a season; it promoted basic science more rapidly being put into practice and was termed "translational medicine." Nevertheless, we see medical communication still has gaps. This chapter will inform the reader what is of importance that may have failed to make the break concerning medication usage.

WAYS TO TAKE MEDICATIONS

Medicines can be taken by mouth (swallowed or held under the tongue), inhaled, injected with a hypodermic needle, or, *gasp* (mostly from children), by rectal suppository. Obviously, injections are the fastest to work followed closely by inhaled or under-the-tongue methods.

One-third of adults experience difficulty when swallowing solid meds.[2] Obviously, moving the meds to the very back of the tongue and dispatching them with a large gulp of liquid helps. A study on the best way to swallow meds showed that relief is obtained by extending the neck forward during swallowing or sucking bottled water from its bottle when swallowing solid meds.[3]

Swallowed meds, however, in order to be effective, depend on the particular medication's absorption curve. Obviously, medications inside the bowel are not active until absorbed. Since most medicine's beneficial actions depend on having a proper amount in the bloodstream (therapeutic range), knowing about the time it takes to reach beneficial levels and how long beneficial levels last is important and we will spend time on that aspect. In general, meds that need to be taken infrequently are absorbed more slowly but also they are eliminated more slowly.

Taking meds once daily is advantageous because the chance of forgetting a dose is reduced. These meds are extended-release and usually are designated as ER on the label.

AVOIDING ADVERSE DRUG REACTIONS

Meds always have problems termed "side effects" or if severe enough, are termed as "adverse drug reactions." Adverse drug reactions are by definition severe enough to require a trip to receive medical care. Side effects are results that are different than the medicine is designed to produce. They usually are not dangerous with one exception—allergic reactions. Allergic reactions range from itchy rashes to having the face swell to difficulty breathing. Having difficulty breathing is the most dangerous; swelling of the face or tongue with difficulty breathing needs an immediate 911 call. Your life is in the balance but an injection, which every paramedic has in their medicine bag, can reverse the process almost immediately.

Adverse drug reactions are more common in elderly patients. In medical lingo, elderly means the transition between middle age and old age (i.e., over 65 years). Adverse reactions serious enough to be reported in Italy were 1.2% annually in persons over 65 years.[4] Unreported reactions are likely many times higher. In one large study, almost 7% of elderly hospital admissions were to treat adverse drug reactions.[5]

Drugs have many side effects; look at the warning sheets included with your prescription. Wow. Those materials are not too helpful because they include many possibilities that are unlikely but are included because of legal consequences. Get information from your doctor. When a new medicine is prescribed, ask, "What should I look out for that would indicate side effects?" The best information, however, is from the pharmacist for what reactions new meds might have because that is their area of expertise.

WHICH ARE THE DANGEROUS DRUGS?

A few drugs are inherently dangerous, such as blood thinners, chemotherapy meds, and antiarrhythmics (meds to keep the heartbeat regular). Patients on dangerous drugs should follow instructions carefully and learn all they can about the medicine from their doctor and reliable sites on the internet. Reliable sources are the Agency for Healthcare Research and Quality (http://www.ahrq.gov/patients-consumers/diagnosis-treatment/treatments/btpills/btpills.html), WebMD, and websites of academic institutions, such as Mayo Clinic and Johns Hopkins.

Dangerous drugs have little flexibility between the dose for the desired effect and the level that causes problems. Blood thinners are prescribed to prevent clotting but can cause bleeding when too much of an effect results. Chemotherapy medications are given to destroy cancer cells which grow faster than normal. But if the effect is too great, chemotherapy medications can damage other fast-dividing cells in the bone marrow and cause the immune system to malfunction. The heartbeat is very sensitive and medications to readjust must be given in the proper doses and the dose between correcting a problem and causing one is narrow. Doctors prescribing dangerous drugs must carefully manage them.

DRUG INTERACTIONS

The most common serious adverse reactions are from drug interactions. The elderly often take a number of medicines because of multiple co-morbidities. One study had the average number of meds for 70-year-olds at eight![3] And the greater the number of meds, the greater is the chance of interactions. Taking too many meds is termed "polypharmacy" and a movement is underway to reduce the number of meds in the elderly with polypharmacy.[6] At least on your yearly checkup visit with your primary care doctor, you should review your meds to make sure you still need each one. On a cautionary note, discontinuing some meds often needs to be gradual because of possible adverse reactions from sudden discontinuance.

As the number of prescribing physicians increase, so do adverse drug reactions.[7] Each additional prescriber increased the chance of adverse effects by almost a third. The problem is a lack of effective communication between prescribers. You, the patient, need to monitor medication changes.

The first line of defense is to inform your primary care doctor's office, probably through the doctor's assistant, that a new medicine is being added by another doctor. That will assure that the doctor that is organizing your overall care is up-to-date. Next, you need to check for drug interactions. Yes, your doctor should have examined your drug list and the pharmacy is supposed to do that but you should always play it safe. In my medical practice, I always wanted to practice cautiously. Try to use one pharmacy, so they will have a complete list of your meds. Several websites have interaction checkers, which work well; WebMD and Walgreens are two.

Years ago, I was boarding a plane to lecture at a medical conference when my cell phone rang. It was Mom who wanted me to know she loved me because she was about to die. This was highly irregular because Mom was one of the most stoic people I knew. I immediately retrieved my luggage, drove 200 miles to Tulsa, and found Mom was correct; she had a pulse rate in the thirties and was about to die from heart failure. She was overmedicated inappropriately with two similar heart meds, which had slowed her pulse rate to disastrous levels. I stopped her meds and by late afternoon, she was feeling much better. I took her to the best restaurant in Tulsa for dinner. I called her doctor, informed him of the overmedication, and requested that I be informed of future medication changes. He was not a happy camper, but agreed. Mom kept seeing him because he was so nice. What? It is nice to have a doctor you like but that is not a good solitary criterion, as mentioned in the chapter on how medicine works.

Instead, judge your doctor by professionalism and results. The doctor should be aware of what you are taking just as you should. I fired a financial advisor because he did not know what my portfolio contained during our conversations. How can advisors advise without knowing your particulars? Review your meds in detail with your doctor when new meds are added or otherwise at least yearly.

Make no mistake: *You are responsible for monitoring your meds.* Bring all of your medicines to each doctor visit. Include any supplements you are taking, so the doctor will be accurately aware of your therapeutic routine. Acts showing you take your therapy seriously will make your doctor more attentive. I almost failed auto shop class in high school but whenever I was told I need auto repairs before wealthy enough to buy a new car, I would ask for explanations of why this needed to be fixed and more often than not, a cheaper alternative was offered.

KEEP A LIST OF MEDICINES

During emergencies, knowledge of medications taken is important. Keeping a list of medicines you and your spouse (or others if you provide their care) take in your wallet or on your smartphone is a safeguard to provide important information if needed and have your spouse do the same.

Medication errors are more common than patients realize. A few years ago, when I was prescribed a rare drug (an antiarrhythmic), a middle practitioner, wrote for a dose that would have soon become an overdose problem. When I pointed it out, she was very embarrassed. The pharmacist would have almost certainly caught the glaring mistake but the point is we must remain on guard. Had I not been a physician, I would not have known the dose was wrong. To guard against errors, patients should know the major side effects of new medications, which is a second layer of protection because overdosing would be likely to have side effects.

Patients have responsibilities at the pharmacy as well. Make sure that the name on the medicine vial is yours. Most of the time the pharmacist will meet with you before you get new meds; if not, ask to meet with the pharmacist.

They should be good at telling you what the medicine is for, what it does, and what side effects it has. Pharmacists are trained specifically about medicines and their nuances.

WHEN TO TAKE MEDICINES

As mentioned at the beginning of this chapter, when to take meds is rarely included with prescriptions. The drug labels tell you how many times a day to swallow them and occasionally advise you to take some with meals. However, our bodies have clocks that synchronize with sleep/wakefulness cycles. For instance, statins that lower our cholesterol work by inhibiting the liver from making it. Our livers make the most cholesterol as we sleep; therefore statins are most effective when taken after the evening meal until bedtime. Cholesterol is necessary but not in excess; it is the foundational molecule to make a number of hormones, especially adrenal steroids and sex hormones. However, it is almost impossible, even with the most powerful statins, to lower cholesterol to a level that interferes with hormone production.

Next, especially with once a day meds, there is a drug concept that is important—drug absorption curve. Low-dose aspirin is glazed with a retardant to keep it from dissolving in the stomach and causing erosions, which can bleed. They are labeled "enteric-coated" or "safety-coated." Enteric-coated, low-dose tablets are the recommended aspirins to take for well-being. Their major function is to prevent heart attacks, among other benefits, by partly disrupting the clotting mechanism. The optimal time to achieve the highest level of aspirin in the morning is to take aspirin at night.[8] Taking coated aspirin at night makes sense because the greatest numbers of heart attacks and the most serious ones occur in the morning hours.[9]

Medicines for high blood pressure consistently have better results when taken at bedtime rather than in the morning.[10] In one study, patients were followed for over five years on the same blood pressure meds with one group taking the meds in the morning and the other at night.[11] The nighttime group had vascular deaths and major vascular events such as heart attacks and strokes that were one-third of the morning group.

People having arthritis pain should note when they have the worst episodes and time their Nonsteroidal anti-inflammatory drugs (NSAID) pain meds four to six hours before. Usually this means the arthritis meds should be taken in the mornings.

As mentioned, medicines that are taken once a day are termed "extended-release" (ER). Many meds are available in ER form. Usually, that is the more desirable form because their absorption and reduction are slower than meds that must be taken more often. Taken less often, they should be taken more regularly. I asked my doctor to arrange my meds so that I take them all once a day. ER meds concentration is lowest just after being taken. As a group, ER meds should be taken at night because metabolism and a lot of risks decrease as we sleep.

As an exception, there are meds that should be taken with meals and others that should be taken on an empty stomach. It does not always hold true but a rule often applies that if the medication should be taken with meals, the pharmacist will place a label advising so on the prescription. If no label is present, take the medicine on an empty stomach, unless it upsets your stomach. Pain meds are rarely labeled because they usually are taken as needed, but some, especially narcotics, should be taken with food to avoid an upset stomach.

ADOPT MEASURES TO ASSURE YOU TAKE YOUR MEDS

Non-compliance is common in the elderly. One can forget to take meds or forget they have taken meds. A Pill Organizer will help prevent this. Develop a routine to ensure compliance. Just before going to turning off the lights and going to bed, I need to do three things: set up coffee, get nightly water poured, and take meds. I leave the medicine containers on the counter when taken to assure me the next morning that they were taken. Establish a routine to take meds and stick to it. Pair it with other repetitive tasks so each reinforces the other. Also, your "smartphone" can be helpful in reminding when to take meds as a backup.

There are some foods that should be avoided when taking certain medicines. When taking blood thinners, one should memorize that considerable list of potentially harmful foods and supplements.

Grapefruit interacts with a number of meds.[12] Particularly, grapefruit affects the absorption of cholesterol-lowering meds and some heart meds and may raise their levels in the blood dangerously high. If you are taking those meds, it would be wise to substitute other citrus and avoid grapefruit altogether.

The liver and kidneys eliminate medications; medications don't just disappear. People with diseases of these organs likely will need to have doses reduced. When getting new prescriptions, patients with decreased function of these organs should remind the prescriber by saying, "Does this dosage take my kidney or liver problems into account?"

COST SAVINGS

Pharmaceutical companies have been brilliant in the last century in giving doctors great tools to treat age-related diseases. The average lifespan in a century has gained almost 50% (24) years (52 years to 76 years) and it has been in no small part from advances in medications. The advances are not cheap; every decade the cost of medical technology has doubled. Patent protections provide the economic impetus to invest huge amounts of money in research. Patent protection lasts 17 years, and then companies other than the developer can apply to produce competitive products, termed "generic medications." Generic means without a trade name; generic is the chemical name.

Recently pharmaceutical companies have been scrimping on development and deplorably have been buying small companies and raising the prices of essential medicines by factors of 500%. This clearly is extortion of vulnerable sick people and must be stopped.

The pharmaceutical and medical device companies have a great system of direct marketing to physicians. They send out drug reps in large numbers who go directly to the medical offices and clinics to convince the doctors that their company's product is better. Pharmaceutical companies are business companies; they promote more expensive medicines, not less expensive ones. They often come bearing gifts. The unwary prescribers (physicians, nurse practitioners, and physician assistants) can be misled into costing their patients more for treatments with no added benefit. Ask your prescriber whether there is a generic that will be as good. The medical profession is generally very professional but there are a number of bumps in the road.

Another pharmaceutical marketing ploy is direct to patient advertising. TV ads are replete with smiling happy people because of buying expensive meds. Remember the past cigarette ads? If you get interested in asking your doctor for the medicine—do it in the manner of asking for an opinion as whether the medicine you are considering will be worth a premium. There are studies showing that patients asking for a specific medicine or test often get it. Remember Garth Brook's song being grateful for "Unanswered Prayers." That is what most of the advertised drugs are about.

Generic drugs cost 20% or even less than brand named ones because they don't share the cost of development. Are generic users settling for less quality? No, not at all. The Food and Drug Administration (FDA) has stringent criteria for approval of generic medications. The chemical composition of active ingredients must be identical and the absorption must be the same. This means the drug works the same way and is in the same amount in the blood stream. Over 2,000 generic's absorptions were compared to the brand's and the generics averaged 96.5%, which provides the same clinical results as the brand name.[13] Further, in dozens of medical studies, outcomes were compared and in every case study were identical.[14]

The FDA monitors both classes of medications for adverse events the same to ensure continued quality. Most non-generic drugs have alternatives in the same class, which will suffice. There are diabetes meds that have no generics to do what they do. A possible difference is that generics may have different additives, other than the active ingredients, than the brand names, which can upset a few patients. Overall, there are few if any reasons for paying premiums for the same drug and the FDA, arguably the most strict federal agency, assures patients it is identical to the more expensive counterpart.

Another area of possible savings is in getting a prescription for an over-the-counter medicine if you take it on a regular basis. A person taking Prilosec at 40 mg daily pays more than a $5 prescription for a month's coverage of the same active ingredient. Getting a prescription for this rather than over the counter is a yearly savings of $345. If you are requiring higher doses of non-narcotics pain relievers such as Aleve or Advil, there are modest savings with prescriptions. Get informed and be involved.

Tablet splitting can cut your cost for medications in half but several steps are necessary to ensure safety. Some time-release medicines and capsules are not eligible for splitting. Tablets that are FDA approved for splitting will say so in the package insert and most will be scored. Some tablets may be split that are not FDA-approved to split; ask your health-care professional. Use a pill splitter and do not split the entire bottle because split tablets can deteriorate faster over time. Do not split tablets that disintegrate; you can't be sure of the dosage.

Generally, larger quantities of the same medicines are cheaper. The standard amount is monthly but medicines taken long-term can be purchased for 90 days—cheaper. And it saves the extra trouble of remembering refills and extra trips. Simplify, simplify, and simplify for a better life.

ARE YOU SUBSIDIZING BIG PHARMA?

Lastly, everything unfortunately expires, including drugs, both prescription drugs and OTC (over-the-counter) meds. A 1979 law required all pharmaceutical and OTC producers to label their products with a date before which they would guarantee potency. Guess what? Their incentive is to sell you medicine. Sounds like the proverbial fox guarding the henhouse.

The military stockpiles a large amount of medicine in case it rapidly becomes needed and they became concerned about the cost of expiration dates. They commissioned a study by the FDA to determine how long meds actually lasted. The study showed almost all meds were just as good as when manufactured after 15 years![15] Another report examined potencies of over 3,000 lots of 122 medications to see if different time of manufacture made a difference. They found that the average time beyond the expiration dates before any drop in potency could be detected was over 5½ years.[16] Much more impressive, a researcher found 14 meds that were expired 28–40 years in a retail pharmacy in original, unopened containers. When these meds were tested for potency, strength was maintained to at least 90% levels of the original prescription.[17] There is a general consensus among experts that storing meds in the refrigerator further extends usefulness.

There are a few exceptions to ignoring the out-of-date dates: nitroglycerin, insulin, and liquid meds. Tetracycline, the antibiotic, questionably becomes toxic. However, the tetracycline toxicity was from a discontinued preparation and no other reports of harm from taking outdated drugs are available.[18] Have we all been throwing away perfectly good meds because we are being fed lies?—no, because we are not informed, which is what we need to make correct choices.

An additional consideration that I have is taking medicine newly on the market on a long-term basis. In Canada, about one-fourth of newly released medications are recalled because of side effects.[11] If a medicine has been on the market for years, I am reassured that long-term use is safe, which is another benefit of generics. They have been available for over a decade which is the patent's protection (20 years) minus the time for Federal Food and Drug Administration approval..

I have always believed that when others embraced the premise that working harder or longer would bring success was true but the real secret to success was working smarter. The same applies to your health choices. Absolutely.

Chapter 17

Everything You Wanted to Know about Supplements But Didn't Know Who to Ask

THE SKINNY ON SUPPLEMENTS

More than half of adult Americans take supplements with the expectation that they will benefit. In one study, 61% of seniors took supplements, which two-thirds started without consulting a medical professional.[1] Half of the subjects thought they had a good effect from over-the-counter supplements and over half did not know whether they had experienced untoward effects or not because they weren't aware of what to expect. The goal of this chapter is to take the mystery out of supplements.

Sometimes if one believes something will benefit, it often does even when it shouldn't.

Not just vitamin stores have nutritional supplements; every grocery store has plentiful supplies. This is because nutritional supplements are a multibillion-dollar industry—about 18 billion in the last count. And on the positive side, people taking supplements lead healthier lifestyles.[2] However, I submit that the supplement-takers are not necessarily leading healthier lifestyles because of supplements. They are likely more conscious of keeping their health and are motivated to do more but that is an opinion.

It is not widely appreciated that whatever supplements you take are of no value whatsoever if not absorbed. Meals gear the body's absorptive mechanisms up a notch, so most supplements should be taken with meals. Mealtime signals the body to release stomach acid and digestive enzymes. In addition, a theoretical advantage is that nutrients, especially antioxidants, in food are clearly superior and taking them with meals seems advantageous. Taking nutrient supplements with meals is not universally determined scientifically but seems a good rule of thumb.

Also, since benefit cannot take place without absorption, absorption cannot take place unless the supplement is available where absorption takes place. Most absorption of meds and supplements takes place in the upper small bowel. The lower small bowel and colon reabsorbs GI secretions and water. For that reason, I prefer capsules to tablets in supplements. Capsules usually dissolve more rapidly and release contents more completely. That is opinion.

However, dissolving is not the primary criterion about which we should be concerned. The amount of absorption of internal meds into the blood stream is the real test. Tests comparing the absorption from nutritional formulations is scant but some studies show capsular form is superior.[3] This question of absorption does not apply to prescriptive meds because the FDA carefully tests their absorption. The pharmaceutical industry recognizes that many consider capsules superior as I do and manufacture caplets—tablets shaped like capsules. They must think minimal of our mentation.

ARE SUPPLEMENTS WELL REGULATED?

These substances are widely taken, sketchily regulated, and have broad health claims that are mostly unproven. "Unlike prescription drugs, dietary supplements do not require premarket review or approval by the FDA. Supplement manufacturers are responsible for determining that their products are safe and their label claims are truthful and not misleading—another fox guarding the henhouse. And, in addition, manufacturers are not required to provide that evidence to the FDA before marketing their products. Wow! If the FDA finds a supplement to be unsafe, it may remove the product from the market or ask the manufacturer to voluntarily recall the product."[4] "FDA regulates both finished dietary supplement products and dietary ingredients. . . . Under the Dietary Supplement Health and Education Act of 1994 (DSHEA)."[5]

Thus, let the buyer beware ("Caveat Emptor") when taking supplements is a wise tact. Going into a supplement store is like going into a used car lot. This is especially true with concoctions for specific health needs, which have multiple substances. Broad unproven categories include men's health, women's health, and brain health. The average supplement for a specific health need has ten ingredients and one I came across in a vitamin shop had over ninety! Interactions with other meds increase as the number of active substances increases. As mentioned, it is a general rule in medicine that when people are taking over six medications, you cannot be sure what the interactions will be. We must assume that holds for chemically active supplements as well, especially if one is taking additional prescription medicines. Interactions of supplements with prescriptive medications can happen. Some of the most commonly taken herbal supplements have undesirable side effects with prescription medications; a top offender is St. John's wort.[6] St. John's wort has a number of interactions with cancer, cardiovascular, and blood thinning medications. People taking blood thinners and cancer medicines should probably avoid herbal supplements altogether, unless cleared with their doctor.

There are a number of herbal supplements, especially St. John's wort, that may interact with blood thinners and blood pressure meds. It is wise for people on blood thinners to avoid herbal supplements and to know what foods to also avoid. Over a decade, blood thinners such as Warfarin, also known as Coumadin, can have serious bleeding episodes in about 20% of patients.

The FDA is a reliable source of information located at its website entitled "Tips for Older Dietary Supplement Users" (http://www.fda.gov/Food/DietarySupplements/UsingDietarySupplements/ucm110493.htm). The bottom line is:

- Dietary supplements are intended to supplement the diet, not to cure, prevent, or treat diseases or replace the variety of foods important to a healthful diet.
- Supplements can help you meet daily requirements for certain nutrients, but when you combine drugs and foods, too much of some nutrients can also cause problems.
- Many factors play a role in deciding if a supplement is right for you, including possible drug interactions and side effects.
- Do not self-diagnose any health condition. Together, you and your healthcare team can make the best decision for optimal health.

Most supplements do not improve the conditions they are thought to improve and perceived benefits are likely from the placebo effect. The placebo effect is pervasive and real enough so that scientific studies are classified as "controlled" by comparing groups given medicine to groups given non-active substances. Those given placebos are in the control group to take the placebo effect into account. It can improve as much as 30% of those given inactive meds.

Another consideration is to be discriminating when you are considering taking supplements, or medications for that matter, long term. It is wise to stop all non-essential supplements for several weeks before elective surgery.

Consumer Reports has identified a "dirty dozen" of supplements that are for sale in America, which have been shown to have dangerous side effects. "The dozen are aconite, bitter orange, chaparral, colloidal silver, coltsfoot, comfrey, country mallow, germanium, greater celandine, kava, lobelia, and yohimbe. The FDA has warned about at least eight of them, some as long ago as 1993."[7] The FDA has not removed potentially harmful supplement ingredients in over a decade. So, it is wise to check the ingredients before taking a supplement long-term and be especially careful with concoctions that have multiple ingredients.

From the huge numbers of herbal supplements taken, it is surprising that interactions with medications are rare. This probably is because most supplements are inert and thus don't have the ability to react.

Since cellular oxidative damage has been shown to be associated with chronic disease, scientists considered that supplemental antioxidants would be protective.[8] However, when multiple studies were combined so that over 100,000 subjects were included, chronic supplementation with beta-carotene, vitamin E, and vitamin A caused an increase in overall mortality, not a decrease as anticipated.[9]

When this and other studies showed a danger in supplemental augmentation of certain antioxidants, I stopped taking them and the multivitamins containing them. In addition, subjects in another study were given 10 of the most popular health supplements for 24 weeks and no improvements in their markers of health were found.[10] It is interesting that ingesting antioxidant-rich foods is health-promoting, whereas obtaining the same substances through supplements is not. The reason for this discrepancy is unclear. There could be unknown cofactors in food but it is clear that food, not supplements, has the greatest benefit.

While there is doubt about ingestion of additional nutrients that have been shown to be beneficial in food, there is no doubt that deficiencies of essential nutrients are harmful. The approach that seems most productive seems to be avoiding deficiencies that occur in the elderly (elderly does not mean old; it means past middle age).

WHAT ABOUT NUTRITIONAL SUPPLEMENTS?

Broadly, your body's nutrient handling consists of three phases: absorption, processing, and elimination. The overall absorption of nutrients is termed "digestion." Digestion is a very efficient process but there is an important point that should be obvious but must be stressed: digestion can only offer the body nutrients that can be broken down from foods that are eaten. In marked contrast to plants, animal bodies, especially the complex higher animal bodies, do not manufacture their life substance from scratch; the molecules composing animal tissues and organs are reassembled from plant and other animal tissues. This means that what humans consume is vital to supply the body's needs. This is especially true for vitamins. Nutritional supplements are added substances that are normally consumed in one's diet.

Among nutritional supplements, some are essential; others, the majority, can be manufactured by the body. As previously mentioned, human bodies need to consume thirteen vitamins, two essential fatty acids (from fat), eight essential amino acids (from protein), and sixteen necessary minerals.

As we age, several factors may cause deficiencies in essential nutrients. Five to ten percent of the elderly are malnourished and a much higher number have nutrient deficiencies.[11] First, older people may not consume diets as varied as they did when younger because of a variety of reasons. Also, elderly bodies may not absorb nutrients as well as when younger.

The least amount of various nutrients that are needed is written on packaged foods as minimum daily requirements. In general, varied diets will adequately supply the minimum daily requirements of essential nutrients. Moderation and diversification as in the stock market investment policy for success is for the most part the secret of a healthy diet. Foods differ in the building blocks and minerals they contain and variation of consumption is necessary.

A Dutch prison doctor, Christiaan Eijkman, noticed chickens fed exclusively prisoner food, which was totally polished rice, staggered like sick prisoners with beriberi; eureka, vitamins were discovered. When fed brown rice, both groups recovered. The husks contain thiamin or vitamin B1.

Currently, the public concept of dietary health regarding vitamins is "more is better." More in biology is not always better. Enough is better in biology. Vitamins and minerals can be taken in excess and produce illness instead of being more healthy.

Vitamins are of two types: water-soluble and fat-soluble. Virtually everything that dissolves in water can be excreted by the kidneys. Nine vitamins dissolve in water and four vitamins dissolve in fats. When excess unneeded water-soluble vitamins are ingested, they are eliminated in urine, so water-soluble vitamins have a safety net—the kidneys, so long as the kidneys are functioning normally. Fat-soluble vitamins cannot be urinated away; they must be metabolized and besides they accumulate in fatty body tissues. Toxic levels produce diseases termed hyper (too much)-vitamin-oses (illnesses).

Remember, –oses designate diseases not caused by infections. Fat-soluble vitamins can be remembered by the phrase, "eek watch out for the DEAK," meaning vitamins D, E, A, and K must be taken in guarded amounts. As we will see, vitamin D is sometimes the exception; even varied diets may be deficient, especially in the elderly.

Vitamin D levels were low indicating deficiency in 90% of elderly community-dwelling French adults.[12] Vitamin D is recognized as a major factor in maintaining healthy bones but it also influences brain function and deficiency may also result in hypertension or depression. In a large study, vitamin D supplements promoted longevity.[10] During an NIH-sponsored conference Dr. Michael Holick, Boston University School of Medicine, Boston, Massachusetts, "gave an overview of vitamin D and discussed the importance of maintaining an adequate vitamin D status." He also reviewed the effects of an inadequate status on a number of different disease states. Vitamin D is known to be important to the maintenance of bone health, as well as playing a role in the prevention of cancers, hypertension, and a number of other diseases common to the elderly. Vitamin D deficiency is very common in U.S. adults, and approximately 50% of the free living and institutionalized elderly are vitamin D deficient, in his opinion.

Also, Vitamin D is important in enhancing the absorption of calcium, inhibiting abnormal cellular growth, and activating both T and B-lymphocytes (important in immunity) function. And is believed to the act in the body's renal system in regard to regulation blood pressure.

A vitamin D deficiency may lead to osteoporosis, and cancer of the colon, prostate, breast, and ovaries. It seems wise to take vitamin D supplements but too much can have bad side effects. WebMD recommends a thousand units a day as a supplement. I take 1,000 units Monday, Wednesday, and Friday— along with B12, folic acid, and thiamin.

Vitamin B12 is another vitamin often found lacking in the elderly. Deficiency ranges from 20% in those over 65 years[13] to about 90% in octogenarians. B12 is necessary for red blood cell production and brain health. B12 is unique in several ways. It is contained in animal protein, not plants, thus, vegans need to supplement. It is rendered absorbable by stomach acid and a protein secreted in the stomach called intrinsic factor, both of which may be insufficient in the elderly. Those taking medicines to reduce stomach acid are especially vulnerable. Notably, deficiencies of B12 need to be administered directly by injection or under the tongue preparations (sublingual) because the problem is absorption, not intake.

Folic acid cannot be synthesized by the human body and must be obtained in the diet. It has very important functions in the synthesis of DNA. This means folic acid is very important in cell replenishment. Folate is normally considered identical to folic acid, especially in supplement labeling, but that is not true. A label of folate may contain multiple related substances. One should take a folic acid preparation.

Folic acid deficiency may cause a sore tongue, diarrhea, depression, confusion, and when severe a specific anemia. Supplements certainly are indicated in pregnant women and the elderly. In a large analysis of multiple studies, scientists found that depression in the elderly was more common in those with low folic acid and B12 levels.[14] Both have no side effects taken in the recommended doses; supplementation has advantages with no appreciable downside.

The most common cause of thiamin deficiency is drinking alcohol.[15] This happens because alcohol interferes with thiamin absorption. Drinking alcohol can lower vitamin B levels, especially thiamin, and supplemental thiamin several times a week is recommended if you imbibe.

Like vitamins, minerals can be taken in excess or be deficient; "the more is better" concept is wrong in supplementation of minerals—definitely. Minerals, except for heavy metals, are easily eliminated by the kidneys, which have exquisitely sensitive methods to keep the concentrations within narrow limits. People with kidney disease must be careful about mineral intake. The major minerals are healthy only within narrow limits.

Potassium may be lost in excess when taking water pills and extra potassium should be taken or abnormal heart rhythms can develop. Contrarily, potassium in excess makes the heart stop. Potassium is the electrolyte injected for executions. With normal kidney function, excess is eliminated in the urine. One must be careful about potassium when kidney function is impaired.

Health is optimized by sufficient intake of the simple substances of life, which besides water includes electrolytes, generally referred to as salts. There are four key electrolytes: sodium (in common table salt), calcium residing in bones, potassium residing in cells, and magnesium.

As mentioned, almost a half century ago a landmark study was done in the isolated Cook Islands located in the South Pacific. My bride and I visited the capital island, Rarotonga, and took a bus ride completely around the island; it took less than an hour. The capital island has had trade with international shipping for centuries and has a "western" diet. Their diet was compared with an isolated island without "western" influence. That island (Pukapuka, I did not make that name up) can only be reached by outrigger boats. The average salt intake was significantly higher on the westernized island where, just as in western locales, blood pressure rose steadily as people aged. On the isolated, salt-restricted island blood pressures remained low into the 70s.[16] In all of medical science, nowhere is it as clearly shown that lifestyle contributes to aging's diseases.

One large study looked at both sodium and potassium intakes and longevity. They followed thousands of subjects for over 14 years and noted higher sodium intakes had higher mortality, whereas higher potassium intakes had lower mortality rates.[17] The differences were particularly striking in the number of deaths from heart disease, which were doubled in those with high sodium and low potassium intakes. Potassium is higher in fruits and veggies, which may account for it appearing to promote health.

Magnesium is the fourth most prevalent electrolyte in human bodies and the only one that is not adequately supplied by many diets. American diets are mostly inadequate to prevent chronic magnesium deficiencies. Overall one-fourth of diets are insufficient in magnesium and this increases to 80% in the elderly.[18] Magnesium is added by eating a variety of nuts, seeds, herbs, and grains that may not be commonly included in American diets: Brazil nuts, molasses, rice, and dark chocolate are examples.

Magnesium is not commonly ordered in laboratory tests as are the other three most common positive electrolytes. Magnesium is necessary for optimal functioning of over three hundred essential biochemical reactions. It promotes muscle, nerve, and bone health. Magnesium stabilizes the heart rhythm, provides reactions for a healthy immune system, and keeps bone tissue strong. Deficiencies have been linked to cardiovascular disease, high blood pressure, diabetes, sudden death syndrome, migraine headaches, muscle cramps, and increased colon cancer. Further, higher intake of magnesium has been shown to reduce colon and rectal cancer.[19]

Magnesium excretion is increased when taking diuretics or drinking alcohol. One or two 400 mg capsules of magnesium daily will supply adequate amounts. It is available in a variety of forms and I recommend magnesium aspartate. When starting supplementation, loose stools may occur, so it is best to take the capsules in the morning with breakfast. Loose stools usually stop with time as the body becomes used to the increased dose.

We all would like to find the perfect antiaging pill but there is none, or is there? Dihydroepiandrosterone (DHEA) is a building block for both male and female hormones. Men and especially women spend a good bit of advanced adult life with lowered hormones. DHEA is a precursor molecule that the body can easily make into sexual hormones. DHEA decreases with aging by 2–5% yearly and is lowered in a number of diseases of aging, including loss of muscle, reduced strength, depression, and possibly Alzheimer's disease. It is important to note that bone density is increased with higher DHEA levels.[20]

Supplementation of DHEA should be at 25 mg to 50 mg daily to provide many potential benefits.[21] These benefits include reduction of muscle loss, improved sexuality, better self-image, reduction in depression, and possible reduction in dementia.

It was of course a marketing tool, but recent scientific studies are favorable, and one day it may rate being called the "fountain of youth" once again.

Chapter 18

Planning a Good Finale

WHAT IS DEATH?

Everyone knows about the made-up aspects of death but it remains the greatest of life's mysteries; is it a beginning, ending, or both? Death, most simply defined, is the permanent unalterable cessation of material consciousness, which makes it the most frightening encounter we have. I was involved with jousting the reaper for almost a half century. The concept of death overwhelms because it could be the end of one's selfhood; as such, it is the ultimate ego affront. Religion's main goal is to reassure that death is not finality for the self.

However, death is inevitable. Thus, all will die. Only two Old Testament men, Enoch and Elijah, and a handful of Greek gods are believed to not have died. Even if they traversed the abyss between material and non-material realities without crossing the river Styx, no one claims to have repeated the feat in thousands of years (Elijah was last 2,900 years ago).

Thus, all material things having a beginning must have an ending. And human bodies, being material things, must end. Many important relationships change with death. These include legal, social, emotional, and religious, and usher in profound obligational changes. A wife's or husband's status becomes a widow or a widower in an instant. The shock, sadness, and obligations accompanying this event need not be as much a problem as is usually experienced. Each of us has seen loved ones have to cope with an unplanned departure, even when the death was predictable for a long time.

PLANNING FOR A GOOD DEATH

No one wants to discuss death, especially the timing when they can expect to depart this life. Most cannot handle that information but when we will die is not the essential element if one plans ahead.

My grandmother Jones has a wise challenge on her tombstone: "Remember me as you pass by. As you are now so once was I. As I am now so shall you be. Prepare for death and follow me." We are all on the same conveyer belt, traveling, at varying speeds, to the identical ultimate event. Preparation can make a great difference in a number of important areas: emotionally, financially, and in closure for family and friends.

Margie Jenkins, a psychologist, who subspecialized in end-of-life counseling, wrote an excellent book on final preparations entitled *You Only Die Once*. Her challenge was to "prepare for the end of life with grace and gusto." Remarkably, she wrote her book when she was an octogenarian. E. P. Baynes considered that dying was losing life's race with death and penned a suggestion to laugh at death. "Death wins! Bravo! But I laugh in his face, as he noses me out at the wire." Whether or not death is the final chapter of selfhood, all need to come to terms with its reality and prepare for death.

First and foremost, a good death literally means dying under optimal circumstances. Each of us must individually define optimal circumstances but a number of specifics are being at home, at ease, and surrounded by loved ones. Perhaps, the next best good death is going to sleep and not awakening. The odds are against that happening and making the best of less than ideal circumstances requires planning. On a positive footnote, I have sat with dying patients with and without their families and my relatives as they passed, and in each instance the word best describing their demeanor is "tranquility" as they slip into whatever eternity holds. My observations differ from obituary's descriptions of "fighting cancer"; at the end all were serene; they simply passed on.

The last six months of life uses more medical resources than any other six months of life. On average, dozens of doctor visit and 12 days are spent hospitalized in the last six months of life. One study of cancer patients showed that one out of six received chemotherapy with its associated illness in the last two weeks of life.[1]

Dartmouth has collected healthcare data for decades. They found large urban medical centers ran significantly greater end-of-life medical bills. As mentioned, most patients prefer to die at home but over half die in hospitals. About one-third died in ICUs. By contrast about 2.5% of elderly with life-limiting disease were under hospice care. It must be noted that admission to an ICU is a more expensive hospital stay but, more importantly, the ICU environment generally means that all available life-sustaining technology will be employed.

Studies have shown that unmanaged end-of-life situations often end with patients hospitalized and having received more care than they or their families desired. The way to manage this potential problem is with an advance directive which specifies what you want done when you cannot make those decisions. The advance directive is not perfect because it limits treatments when the prognosis is judged to be futile.

Most family members find the decision to limit treatment of a loved one troubling. They do not but should realize that the disease, not their decision to limit care, rationally will cause the death. Completing an advance directive protects them from having to make the painful decision to limit care at a time when they are already distressed.

Physicians, especially surgeons, can at times have difficulty in letting patients go. After all, most seasoned surgeons, especially cardiovascular and trauma surgeons, have seen a few amazing recoveries. Having an advanced directive and specifying who one wants to have the power of attorney makes a difficult situation less stressful on all the participants.

Physicians have completed advance directives in over three times the rate of the general public,[2] and it is surprising that 100% do not have directives, are aware how application of technology can spiral out of control at life's end. Medical care becomes patient and family-controlled, and faced with the reaper, the "do everything mandate" often becomes the driver.

Originally proposed as "living wills," the documents allowing incapacitated patients to decide their medical care have become more popularly called advance directives. They are insurance policies for as good a death as possible. Having been around seriously ill people over a long career, I did not see advance directives being misused. The attending physicians have great respect for the preservation of life and relief of suffering. There is little chance of giving up too early; advance directives stop futile care in hopeless situations.

Although the format is essentially the same, each state's requirements must be met. This is made easy by free forms on the internet or there are websites that for a nominal fee will walk one through your state's form. Each state has a separate but similar form with instructions about what is meant. The Texas form is very well done. It is available at www.caringinfo.org/files/public/ad/Texas.pdf.

The message is clear and agreed to by over 90% of adults: don't continue to keep me alive if doing so cannot return me to a state of meaningful interaction with the environment. I once had a great conflict with a family wanting what I considered early discontinuation of life support in a patient with a dense stroke. Their mantra was "he would not want to live if he couldn't play golf." I had a great deal of trouble with that determination of the worthwhileness of life. The conflict resolved as his condition worsened, becoming futile.

Medical futility is a clear end-point that should summon withdrawal of medical care without regret for family or physician. There are four categories.[3] "Physiologic futility" is recognized when the medical intervention is reliably expected not to produce its desired physiologic effect. Cardiopulmonary resuscitation is routinely discontinued when it can no longer be expected to restore spontaneous circulation and respiration. "Overall futility" reflects a reliable expectation that the intervention will not restore the patient's capacity to interact with the environment and continue human development. Antibiotics for management of opportunistic infections can justifiably be withheld from patients in a persistent vegetative state. "Imminent demise futility" characterizes a reliable expectation that the patient will die before discharge and not recover interactive capacity before death. "Quality of life futility" applies when the patient's current or projected condition will result in an intolerable inability to engage in or derive pleasure from life. The futility concept should be the guide to avoid overtreatment.

Health care is only one of the preparations needed. A standard legal will can make certain that assets go to those you want and avoid unnecessary losses through taxes.

Margie Jenkins's book *You Only Die Once* emphasizes the frequently unappreciated importance of preparing for the second most important day of one's life. Margie's insightful practical suggestions enriched the preparations for my mother's funeral and our end-of-life relationship tremendously. We talked about Mom's feelings about dying. Her words on her death bed still resonate in my mind providing comfort. She said, "I have done everything expected of me. Nothing remains. It is time." She described how she wanted her funeral to be conducted. I had to shop for a white gown and her smile was my reward when I showed her what would clothe her for eternity. She was born in a northern Arkansas town, which is still populated by less than a hundred people. The preacher was honored to conduct her services and she was laid to rest next to Dad.

Mother had Alzheimer's disease and we auctioned most of her goods in an estate sale, keeping only a few mementos. However, I will avoid having some of the things I treasured be sold to strangers by following a suggestion from Margie: each of our children were told to list the things they wanted in order.

Write your epitaph. It will proclaim who you were to all who pass by. Mine is: "Listen, hear God whisper: Forgive, forgive all, Eternity has no anger; Smile, laugh, rejoice, Eternity has no tears; Despair not death's kiss, Eternity restores all."

A good healthy life ending in a good death is the theme of this book.

Notes

INTRODUCTION

1. Lorin, M. I., Palazzi, D. L., Turner, T. L. and Ward, M. A. What is a clinical pearl and what is its role in medical education? *Medical Teacher* 2008; 30: 870–4.

2. Haidt, J. *The Happiness Hypothesis*. New York: Basic Books, Perseus Group, 2006.

CHAPTER 1

1. Herskind, A. M., McGue, M., Holm, N. V., Sorensen, T. I., Harvald, B. and Vaupel, J. W. The heritability of human longevity: a population-based study of 2872 Danish twin pairs born 1870–1900. *Human Genetics* 1996; 97: 319–23.

2. Knoops, K. T., de Groot, L. C., Kromhout, D., et al. Mediterranean diet, lifestyle factors, and 10-year mortality in elderly European men and women: the HALE project. *JAMA* 2004; 292: 1433–9.

3. Stessman, J., Hammerman-Rozenberg, R., Cohen, A., Ein-Mor, E. and Jacobs, J. M. Physical activity, function, and longevity among the very old. *Archives of Internal Medicine* 2009; 169: 1476–83.

4. Loprinzi, P. D., Smit, E. and Mahoney, S. Physical activity and dietary behavior in US adults and their combined influence on health. *Mayo Clinic Proceedings Mayo Clinic* 2014; 89: 190–8.

5. Bostock, S. and Steptoe, A. Association between low functional health literacy and mortality in older adults: longitudinal cohort study. *BMJ* 2012; 344: e1602.

6. Eagleman, D. *Incognito: The Secret Lives of the Brain*. New York: Pantheon Books; 2011.

185

7. Hopkins, M. E., Davis, F. C., Vantieghem, M. R., Whalen, P. J. and Bucci, D. J. Differential effects of acute and regular physical exercise on cognition and affect. *Neuroscience* 2012; 215: 59–68.

8. Windle, G., Hughes, D., Linck, P., Russell, I. and Woods, B. Is exercise effective in promoting mental well-being in older age? A systematic review. *Aging & Mental Health* 2010; 14: 652–69.

9. Rosa, J. P., de Souza, A. A., de Lima, G. H., et al. Motivational and evolutionary aspects of a physical exercise training program: a longitudinal study. *Frontiers in Psychology* 2015; 6: 648.

10. Desplan, M., Mercier, J., Sabate, M., Ninot, G., Prefaut, C. and Dauvilliers, Y. A comprehensive rehabilitation program improves disease severity in patients with obstructive sleep apnea syndrome: a pilot randomized controlled study. *Sleep Medicine* 2014; 8: 906–12.

11. Hsiao, W., Shrewsberry, A. B., Moses, K. A., et al. Exercise is associated with better erectile function in men under 40 as evaluated by the international index of erectile function. *The Journal of Sexual Medicine* 2012; 9: 524–30.

12. Melancon, M. O., Lorrain, D. and Dionne, I. J. Changes in markers of brain serotonin activity in response to chronic exercise in senior men. *Applied Physiology, Nutrition, and Metabolism = Physiologie Appliquee, Nutrition et Metabolisme* 2014; 11: 1250–6.

13. Fattore, L., Fadda, P., Spano, M. S., Pistis, M. and Fratta, W. Neurobiological mechanisms of cannabinoid addiction. *Molecular and Cellular Endocrinology* 2008; 286: S97–107.

14. Jacka, F. N., Mykletun, A., Berk, M., Bjelland, I. and Tell, G. S. The association between habitual diet quality and the common mental disorders in community-dwelling adults: the Hordaland Health study. *Psychosomatic Medicine* 2011; 73 :483–90.

15. Justine, M., Azizan, A., Hassan, V., Salleh, Z. and Manaf, H. Barriers to participation in physical activity and exercise among middle-aged and elderly individuals. *Singapore Medical Journal* 2013; 54: 581–6.

16. Mischel, W., Ebbesen, E. B. and Zeiss, A. R. Cognitive and attentional mechanisms in delay of gratification. *Journal of Personality and Social Psychology* 1972; 21: 204–18.

17. Tate, L. M. Temporal discounting rates and their relation to exercise behavior in older adults. *Physiology & Behavior* 2015; 152: 295–9.

18. Lawyer, S. R., Boomhower, S. R., Rasmussen, E. B. Differential associations between obesity and behavioral measures of impulsivity. *Appetite* 2015; 95: 375–82.

19. Cherkas, L. F., Hunkin, J. L., Kato, B. S., et al. The association between physical activity in leisure time and leukocyte telomere length. *Archives of Internal Medicine* 2008; 168: 154–8.

20. Bendix, L., Gade, M. M., Staun, P. W., et al. Leukocyte telomere length and physical ability among Danish twins age 70+. *Mechanisms of Ageing and Development* 2011; 132: 568–72.

CHAPTER 2

1. Erickson, K. I., Voss, M. W., Prakash, R. S., et al. Exercise training increases size of hippocampus and improves memory. *Proceedings of the National Academy of Sciences of the United States of America* 2011; 108: 3017–22.

CHAPTER 4

1. Leung, C. W., Laraia, B. A., Needham, B. L., et al. Soda and cell aging: associations between sugar-sweetened beverage consumption and leukocyte telomere length in healthy adults from the national health and nutrition eExamination surveys. *American Journal of Public Health* 2014: 12: 2425–31.

2. Speakman, J. R., Selman, C., McLaren, J. S. and Harper, E. J. Living fast, dying when? the link between aging and energetics. *The Journal of Nutrition* 2002; 132: 1583S–97S.

3. Agarwal, S. and Sohal, R. S. DNA oxidative damage and life expectancy in houseflies. *Proceedings of the National Academy of Sciences of the United States of America* 1994; 91: 12332–5.

4. Schols, J. M., de Groot, C. P., van der Cammen, T. J. and Olde Rikkert, M. G. Preventing and treating dehydration in the elderly during periods of illness and warm weather. *The Journal of Nutrition, Health & Aging* 2009; 13: 150–7.

5. Volkert, D., Kreuel, K. and Stehle, P. Fluid intake of community-living, independent elderly in Germany—a nationwide, representative study. *The Journal of Nutrition, Health & Aging* 2005; 9: 305–9.

6. Prior, I. A., Evans, J. G., Harvey, H. P., Davidson, F. and Lindsey, M. Sodium intake and blood pressure in two Polynesian populations. *New England Journal of Medicine* 1968; 279: 515–20.

7. Rosanoff, A., Weaver, C. M. and Rude, R. K. Suboptimal magnesium status in the United States: are the health consequences underestimated? *Nutrition Reviews* 2012; 70: 153–64.

8. Wark, P. A., Lau, R., Norat, T. and Kampman, E. Magnesium intake and colorectal tumor risk: a case-control study and meta-analysis. *The American Journal of Clinical Nutrition* 2012; 93: 622–31

CHAPTER 5

1. Dahlgren, J., Warshaw, R., Thornton, J., Anderson-Mahoney, C. P. and Takhar, H. Health effects on nearby residents of a wood treatment plant. *Environmental Research* 2003; 92: 92–8.

2. Okada, F. Inflammation-related carcinogenesis: current findings in epidemiological trends, causes and mechanisms. *Yonago Acta Medica* 2014; 57: 65–72.

3. Graham, D. Y., Go, M. F. and Genta, R. M. Helicobacter pylori, duodenal ulcer, gastric cancer: tunnel vision or blinders? *Annals of Medicine* 1995; 27: 589–94.

4. Raison, C. L. and Miller, A. H. Is depression an inflammatory disorder? *Current Psychiatry Reports* 2011; 13: 467–75.

5. Diehl, A. K. Review: daily aspirin reduces short-term risk for cancer and cancer mortality. *Annals of Internal Medicine* 2012; 157: JC1–2.

6. Cuzick, J., Thorat, M. A., Andriole, G., et al. Prevention and early detection of prostate cancer. *The Lancet Oncology* 2014; 15: e484–92.

7. Zhang, S., Zhang, X. Q., Ding, X. W., et al. Cyclooxygenase inhibitors use is associated with reduced risk of esophageal adenocarcinoma in patients with Barrett's esophagus: a meta-analysis. *British Journal of Cancer* 2014; 110: 2378–88.

8. Hur, C., Simon, L. S. and Gazelle, G. S. The cost-effectiveness of aspirin versus cyclooxygenase-2-selective inhibitors for colorectal carcinoma chemoprevention in healthy individuals. *Cancer* 2004; 101: 189–97.

9. Gierach, G. L., Lacey, J. V., Jr., Schatzkin, A., et al. Nonsteroidal anti-inflammatory drugs and breast cancer risk in the National Institutes of Health-AARP Diet and Health Study. *Breast Cancer Research* (BCR) 2008; 10: R38.

10. Ibid.

11. Loucks, E. B., Sullivan, L. M., D'Agostino, R. B., Sr., Larson, M. G., Berkman, L. F. and Benjamin. E. J. Social networks and inflammatory markers in the Framingham Heart Study. *Journal of Biosocial Science* 2006; 38: 835–42.

12. Goto, M., Sugimoto, K., Hayashi, S., et al. Aging-associated inflammation in healthy Japanese individuals and patients with Werner syndrome. *Experimental 3* 2012; 47: 936–9.

13. Okada, H. C., Alleyne, B., Varghai, K., Kinder, K. and Guyuron, B. Facial changes caused by smoking: a comparison between smoking and nonsmoking identical twins. *Plastic and Reconstructive Surgery* 2013; 132: 1085–92.

14. Chen, X., Mao, G. and Leng, S. X. Frailty syndrome: an overview. *Clinical Interventions in Aging* 2014; 9: 433–41.

15. Gale, C. R., Baylis, D., Cooper, C. and Sayer, A. A. Inflammatory markers and incident frailty in men and women: the English Longitudinal Study of Ageing. *Age* 2013; 35: 2493–2501.

16. Koenig, W., Khuseyinova, N., Baumert, J. and Meisinger, C. Prospective study of high-sensitivity C-reactive protein as a determinant of mortality: results from the MONICA/KORA Augsburg Cohort Study, 1984–1998. *Clinical Chemistry* 2008; 54: 335–42.

17. Menotti, A., Puddu, P. E., Lanti, M., Maiani, G., Catasta, G. and Fidanza, A. A. Lifestyle habits and mortality from all and specific causes of death: 40-year follow-up in the Italian Rural Areas of the Seven Countries Study. *The Journal of Nutrition, Health & Aging* 2014; 18: 314–21.

18. Hamer, M., Sabia, S., Batty, G. D., et al. Physical activity and inflammatory markers over 10 years: follow-up in men and women from the Whitehall II cohort study. *Circulation* 2012; 126: 928–33.

19. Wang, B., Li, Z., Miao, M. et al. The relationship between physical activity and aging symptoms among community-dwelling men aged 40–70 years in Shanghai, China. *Journal of Physical Activity & Health* 2014; 1: 87-92.

20. Kuczmarski, M. F., Mason, M. A., Allegro, D., Zonderman, A. B. and Evans, M. K. Diet quality is inversely associated with C-reactive protein levels in urban, low-income African-American and white adults. *Journal of the Academy of Nutrition and Dietetics* 2013; 113: 1620–31.

21. Nielsen, F. H., Johnson, L. K. and Zeng, H. Magnesium supplementation improves indicators of low magnesium status and inflammatory stress in adults older than 51 years with poor quality sleep. *Magnesium Research: Official Organ of the International Society for the Development of Research on Magnesium* 2010; 23: 158–68.

22. Noack, B., Genco, R. J., Trevisan, M., Grossi, S., Zambon, J. J. and de Nardin, E. Periodontal infections contribute to elevated systemic C-reactive protein level. *Journal of Periodontology* 2001; 72: 1221–7.

23. Kantor, E. D., Lampe, J. W., Kratz, M. and White, E. Lifestyle factors and inflammation: associations by body mass index. *PLoS ONE* 2013; 8: e67833.

24. Bardia, A., Ebbert, J. O., Vierkant, R. A., et al. Association of aspirin and nonaspirin nonsteroidal anti-inflammatory drugs with cancer incidence and mortality. *Journal of the National Cancer Institute* 2007; 99: 881–9.

25. Hirata, Y., Kataoka, H., Shimura, T., et al. Incidence of gastrointestinal bleeding in patients with cardiovascular disease: buffered aspirin versus enteric-coated aspirin. *Scandinavian Journal of Gastroenterology* 2011; 46: 803–9.

26. Puhan, M. A., Singh, S., Weiss, C. O., Varadhan, R., Sharma, R. and Boyd, C. M. In *Evaluation of the Benefits and Harms of Aspirin for Primary Prevention of Cardiovascular Events: A Comparison of Quantitative Approaches*. Rockville, MD: Agency for Healthcare Research and Quality, 2013.

CHAPTER 6

1. Knoops, K. T., de Groot, L. C., Kromhout, D., et al. Mediterranean diet, lifestyle factors, and 10-year mortality in elderly European men and women: the HALE project. *JAMA* 2004; 292: 1433–9.

2. Trichopoulou, A., Bamia, C. and Trichopoulos, D. Mediterranean diet and survival among patients with coronary heart disease in Greece. *Archives of Internal Medicine* 2005; 165: 929–35.

3. Adams, B. J., Carr, J. G., Ozonoff, A., Lauer, M. S. and Balady, G. J. Effect of exercise training in supervised cardiac rehabilitation programs on prognostic variables from the exercise tolerance test. *American Journal of Cardiology* 2008; 101: 1403–7.

CHAPTER 7

1. Luders, E., Narr, K. L., Bilder, R. M., et al. Mapping the relationship between cortical convolution and intelligence: effects of gender. *Cerebral Cortex* 2008; 18: 2019–26.

2. Inta, D., Cameron, H. A. and Gass, P. New neurons in the adult striatum: from rodents to humans. *Trends in Neurosciences* 2015; 38: 517–23.

3. Erickson, K. I., Prakash, R. S., Voss, M. W., et al. Aerobic fitness is associated with hippocampal volume in elderly humans. *Hippocampus* 2009; 19: 1030–9.

4. Erickson, K. I., Voss, M. W., Prakash, R. S., et al. Exercise training increases size of hippocampus and improves memory. *Proceedings of the National Academy of Sciences of the United States of America* 2011; 108: 3017–22.

5. Bremner, J. D., Narayan, M., Anderson, E. R., Staib, L. H., Miller, H. L. and Charney, D. S. Hippocampal volume reduction in major depression. *The American Journal of Psychiatry* 2000; 157: 115–18.

6. Sterling, D. A., O'Connor, J. A. and Bonadies, J. Geriatric falls: injury severity is high and disproportionate to mechanism. *The Journal of Trauma* 2001; 50: 116–19.

7. Panza, F., D'Introno, A., Colacicco, A. M., et al. Cognitive frailty: pre-dementia syndrome and vascular risk factors. *Neurobiology of Aging* 2006; 27: 933–40.

8. van den Dungen, P., Moll van Charante, E. P., van de Ven, P. M., et al. Dutch family physicians' awareness of cognitive impairment among the elderly. *BMC Geriatrics* 2015; 15: 105.

9. Barnes, D. E., Covinsky, K. E., Whitmer, R. A., Kuller, L. H., Lopez, O. L. and Yaffe, K. Predicting risk of dementia in older adults: the late-life dementia risk index. *Neurology* 2009; 73: 173–9.

10. Yi, H. A., Moller, C., Dieleman, N., et al. Relation between subcortical grey matter atrophy and conversion from mild cognitive impairment to Alzheimer's disease. *Journal of Neurology, Neurosurgery, and Psychiatry* 2015; 87: 425–32.

11. Miller, J. W., Harvey, D. J., Beckett, L. A., et al. Vitamin D status and rates of cognitive decline in a multiethnic cohort of older adults. *JAMA Neurology* 2015; 92: 1295–1303.

12. Jick, H., Zornberg, G. L., Jick, S. S., Seshadri, S. and Drachman, D. A. Statins and the risk of dementia. *Lancet* 2000; 356: 1627–31.

13. Fratiglioni, L., Wang, H. X., Ericsson, K., Maytan, M. and Winblad, B. Influence of social network on occurrence of dementia: a community-based longitudinal study. *Lancet* 2000; 355: 1315–19.

14. Jedrziewski, M. K., Ewbank, D. C., Wang, H. and Trojanowski, J. Q. The impact of exercise, cognitive activities, and socialization on cognitive function: results from the national long-term care survey. *American Journal of Alzheimer's Disease and other Dementias* 2014; 29: 372–8.

15. Paillard, T., Rolland, Y. and de Souto Barreto, P. Protective effects of physical exercise in Alzheimer's disease and Parkinson's disease: a narrative review. *Journal of Clinical Neurology* 2015; 11: 212–9.

16. Abbott, R. D., White, L. R., Ross, G. W., Masaki, K. H., Curb, J. D. and Petrovitch, H. Walking and dementia in physically capable elderly men. *JAMA* 2004; 292: 1447–53.

17. Valls-Pedret, C., Sala-Vila, A., Serra-Mir, M., et al. Mediterranean diet and age-related cognitive decline: a randomized clinical trial. *JAMA Internal Medicine* 2015; 175: 1094–103.

18. Gu, Y., Nieves, J. W., Stern, Y., Luchsinger, J. A. and Scarmeas, N. Food combination and Alzheimer disease risk: a protective diet. *Archives of Neurology* 2010; 67: 699–706.

19. Letenneur, L. Risk of dementia and alcohol and wine consumption: a review of recent results. *Biological Research* 2004; 37: 189–93.

20. Ngandu, T., Lehtisalo, J., Solomon, A., et al. A 2 year multidomain intervention of diet, exercise, cognitive training, and vascular risk monitoring versus control to prevent cognitive decline in at-risk elderly people (FINGER): a randomised controlled trial., *Lancet* 2015; 385: 2255–63.

21. Scarmeas, N., Luchsinger, J. A., Schupf, N., et al. Physical activity, diet, and risk of Alzheimer disease. *JAMA* 2009; 302: 627–37.

CHAPTER 8

1. Bernstein, M. S., Morabia, A. and Sloutskis, D. Definition and prevalence of sedentarism in an urban population. *American Journal of Public Health* 1999; 89: 862–7.

2. Gill, S. S. and Seitz, D. P. Lifestyles and cognitive health: what older individuals can do to optimize cognitive outcomes. *JAMA* 2015; 314: 774–5.

3. Chen, X., Mao, G. and Leng, S. X. Frailty syndrome: an overview. *Clinical Interventions in Aging* 2014; 9: 433–41.

4. Du, M., Prescott, J., Kraft, P., et al. Physical activity, sedentary behavior, and leukocyte telomere length in women. *American Journal of Epidemiology* 2012; 175: 414–22.

5. Balboa-Castillo, T., Guallar-Castillon, P., Leon-Munoz, L. M., Graciani, A., Lopez-Garcia, E. and Rodriguez-Artalejo, F. Physical activity and mortality related to obesity and functional status in older adults in Spain. *American Journal of Preventive Medicine* 2011; 40: 39–46.

6. Windle, G., Hughes, D., Linck, P., Russell, I. and Woods, B. Is exercise effective in promoting mental well-being in older age? A systematic review. *Aging & Mental Health* 2010; 14: 652–69.

7. Sjogren, P., Fisher, R., Kallings, L., Svenson, U., Roos, G. and Hellenius, M. L. Stand up for health—avoiding sedentary behaviour might lengthen your telomeres: secondary outcomes from a physical activity RCT in older people. *British Journal of Sports Medicine* 2014; 48: 1407–9.

8. Fratiglioni, L., Wang, H. X., Ericsson, K., Maytan, M. and Winblad, B. Influence of social network on occurrence of dementia: a community-based longitudinal study. *Lancet* 2000; 355: 1315–19.

9. Gleibs, I. H., Haslam, C., Jones, J. M., Alexander Haslam, S., McNeill, J. and Connolly, H. No country for old men? The role of a 'Gentlemen's Club' in promoting social engagement and psychological well-being in residential care. *Aging & Mental Health* 2011; 15: 456–66.

10. Zuliani, G., Soavi, C., Dainese, A., Milani, P. and Gatti, M. Diogenes syndrome or isolated syllogomania? Four heterogeneous clinical cases. *Aging Clinical and Experimental Research* 2013; 25: 473–8.

11. Maness, D. L. and Khan, M. Nonpharmacologic Management of Chronic Insomnia. *American Family Physician* 2015; 92: 1058–64.

12. Rahe, C., Czira, M. E., Teismann, H. and Berger, K. Associations between poor sleep quality and different measures of obesity. *Sleep medicine* 2015; 16: 1225–8.

13. Mansukhani, M. P., Wang, S. and Somers, V. K. Sleep, death, and the heart. *American Journal of Physiology Heart and Circulatory Physiology* 2015; 309: H739–49.

14. Urban, L. E., Weber, J. L., Heyman, M. B., et al. Energy contents of frequently ordered restaurant meals and comparison with human energy requirements and US department of agriculture database information: a multisite randomized study. *Journal of the Academy of Nutrition and Dietetics* 2016; 116: 590–598.

15. Colman, R. J., Beasley, T. M., Kemnitz, J. W., Johnson, S. C., Weindruch, R. and Anderson, R. M. Caloric restriction reduces age-related and all-cause mortality in rhesus monkeys. *Nature Communications* 2014; 5: 3557.

16. Castro-Quezada, I., Sanchez-Villegas, A., Estruch, R., et al. A high dietary glycemic index increases total mortality in a Mediterranean population at high cardiovascular risk. *PloS One* 2014; 9: e107968.

17. Weihrauch, M. R. and Diehl, V. Artificial sweeteners—do they bear a carcinogenic risk? *Annals of Oncology: Official Journal of the European Society for Medical Oncology/ESMO* 2004; 15: 1460–5.

CHAPTER 9

1. Carlsohn, A., Rohn, S, Bittmann, F., Raila, J., Mayer, F. and Schweigert, F. J. Exercise increases the plasma antioxidant capacity of adolescent athletes. *Annals of Nutrition & Metabolism* 2008; 53: 96–103.

2. Ji, L. L. Exercise at old age: does it increase or alleviate oxidative stress? *Annals of the New York Academy of Sciences* 2001; 928: 236–47.

3. Pleis, J. R., Ward, B. W. and Lucas, J. W. Summary health statistics for U.S. adults: National Health Interview Survey, 2009. Vital and health statistics Series 10, Data from the National Health Survey 2010: 1–207.

4. Paffenbarger, R. S., Jr., Kampert, J. B., Lee, I. M., Hyde, R. T., Leung, R. W. and Wing, A. L. Changes in physical activity and other lifeway patterns influencing longevity. *Medicine and Science in Sports and Exercise* 1994; 26: 857–65.

5. Brown, W. J., McLaughlin, D., Leung, J., et al. Physical activity and all-cause mortality in older women and men. *British Journal of Sports Medicine* 2012; 46: 664–8.

6. Whang, W., Manson, J. E., Hu, F. B., et al. Physical exertion, exercise, and sudden cardiac death in women. *JAMA* 2006; 295: 1399–1403.

7. Leading causes of death. In: http://www.cdc.gov/nchs/fastats/lcod.htm: Centers for Disease Control and Prevention, 2009.

8. Kurl, S., Laukkanen, J. A., Rauramaa, R., Lakka, T. A., Sivenius, J. and Salonen, J. T. Cardiorespiratory fitness and the risk for stroke in men. *Archives of Internal Medicine* 2003; 163: 1682–8.

9. Dahabreh, I. J. and Paulus, J. K. Association of episodic physical and sexual activity with triggering of acute cardiac events: systematic review and meta-analysis. *JAMA* 2011; 305: 1225–33.

10. McCallum, J., Simons, L. A., Simons, J. and Friedlander, Y. Delaying dementia and nursing home placement: the Dubbo study of elderly Australians over a 14-year follow-up. *Annals of the New York Academy Sciences* 2007; 1114: 121–9.

11. Wallace, R., Lees, C., Minou, M., Singleton, D. and Stratton, G. Effects of a 12-week community exercise programme on older people. *Nursing Older People* 2014; 26: 20–6.

12. Artaud, F., Dugravot, A., Sabia, S., Singh-Manoux, A., Tzourio, C. and Elbaz, A. Unhealthy behaviours and disability in older adults: three-City Dijon cohort study. *BMJ* 2013; 347: f4240.

13. Weuve, J., Kang, J. H., Manson, J. E., Breteler, M. M., Ware, J. H. and Grodstein, F. Physical activity, including walking, and cognitive function in older women. *JAMA* 2004; 292: 1454–61.

14. Erickson, K. I., Prakash, R. S., Voss, M. W., et al. Aerobic fitness is associated with hippocampal volume in elderly humans. *Hippocampus* 2009; 19: 1030–9.

15. Erickson, K. I., Voss, M. W., Prakash, R. S., et al. Exercise training increases size of hippocampus and improves memory. *Proceedings of the National Academy of Sciences of the United States of America* 2011; 108: 3017–22.

16. Hopkins, M. E., Davis, F. C., Vantieghem, M. R., Whalen, P. J. and Bucci, D. J. Differential effects of acute and regular physical exercise on cognition and affect. *Neuroscience* 2012; 215: 59–68.

17. Goekint, M., De Pauw, K., Roelands, B., et al. Strength training does not influence serum brain-derived neurotrophic factor. *European Journal of Applied Physiology* 2010; 110: 285–93.

18. Parker, S. J., Strath, S. J. and Swartz, A. M. Physical activity measurement in older adults: relationships with mental health. *Journal of Aging Physical Activity* 2008; 16: 369–80.

19. Balboa-Castillo, T., Guallar-Castillon, P., Leon-Munoz, L. M., Graciani, A., Lopez-Garcia, E. and Rodriguez-Artalejo, F. Physical activity and mortality related to obesity and functional status in older adults in Spain. *American Journal of Preventive Medicine* 2011; 40: 39–46.

20. Greenlees, I. A., Hall, B., Manley, A. and Thelwell, R. C. How older adults are perceived is influenced by their reported exercise status. *Journal of Aging Physical Activity* 2011; 19: 279–90.

21. La Vignera, S., Condorelli, R., Vicari, E., D'Agata, R. and Calogero, A. E. Physical activity and erectile dysfunction in middle-aged men. *Journal of Andrology* 2012; 33: 154–61.

22. Hsiao, W., Shrewsberry, A. B., Moses, K. A., et al. Exercise is associated with better erectile function in men under 40 as evaluated by the international index of erectile function. *The Journal of Sexual Medicine* 2012; 9: 524–30.

23. Cohen, P. A. and Venhuis, B. J. Adulterated sexual enhancement supplements: more than mojo. *JAMA Internal Medicine* 2013; 173: 1169–70.

24. Esposito, K., Giugliano, F., Di Palo, C., et al. Effect of lifestyle changes on erectile dysfunction in obese men: a randomized controlled trial. *JAMA* 2004; 291: 2978–84.

25. Chen, J., Wollman, Y., Chernichovsky, T., Iaina, A., Sofer, M. and Matzkin, H. Effect of oral administration of high-dose nitric oxide donor L-arginine in men with organic erectile dysfunction: results of a double-blind, randomized, placebo-controlled study. *BJU International* 1999; 83: 269–73.

26. Appleton, J. Arginine: Clinical potential of a semi-essential amino acid. *Alternative Medicine Review: A Journal of Clinical Therapeutic* 2002; 7: 512–22.

27. Verma, M., Khoury, M. J. and Ioannidis, J. P. Opportunities and challenges for selected emerging technologies in cancer epidemiology: mitochondrial, epigenomic, metabolomic, and telomerase profiling. *Cancer Epidemiology, Biomarkers & Prevention: A Publication of the American Association for Cancer Research, Cosponsored by the American Society of Preventive Oncology* 2013; 22: 189–200.

28. Du, M., Prescott, J., Kraft, P., et al. Physical activity, sedentary behavior, and leukocyte telomere length in women. *American Journal of Epidemiology* 2012; 175: 414–22.

29. Cherkas, L. F., Hunkin, J. L., Kato, B. S., et al. The association between physical activity in leisure time and leukocyte telomere length. *Archives of Internal Medicine* 2008; 168: 154–8.

CHAPTER 10

1. Fabian, E., Bogner, M., Kickinger, A., Wagner, K. H. and Elmadfa, I. Vitamin status in elderly people in relation to the use of nutritional supplements. *The Journal of Nutrition, Health & Aging* 2012; 16: 206–12.

2. Chei, C. L., Raman, P., Yin, Z. X., Shi, X. M., Zeng, Y. and Matchar, D. B. Vitamin D levels and cognition in elderly adults in China. *Journal of the American Geriatrics Society* 2014; 62: 2125–9.

3. Miller, J. W., Harvey, D. J., Beckett, L. A., et al. Vitamin D status and rates of cognitive decline in a multiethnic cohort of older adults. *JAMA Neurology* 2015; 72: 1295–1303.

4. Karakis, I., Pase, M. P., Beiser, A., et al. Association of Serum Vitamin D with the risk of incident dementia and subclinical indices of brain aging: The Framingham heart study. *Journal of Alzheimer's disease: JAD* 2016; 51: 451–461.

5. Lindenbaum, J., Rosenberg, I. H., Wilson, P. W., Stabler, S. P. and Allen, R. H. Prevalence of cobalamin deficiency in the Framingham elderly population. *The American Journal of Clinical Nutrition* 1994; 60: 2–11.

6. Yang, Q., Liu, T., Kuklina, E. V., et al. Sodium and potassium intake and mortality among US adults: prospective data from the Third National Health and Nutrition Examination Survey. *Archives of Internal Medicine* 2011; 171: 1183–91.

7. Lane, M. A., Black, A., Handy, A., Tilmont, E. M., Ingram, D. K. and Roth, G. S. Caloric restriction in primates. *Annals of the New York Academy of Sciences* 2001; 928: 287–95.

8. Du, D., Shi, Y. H. and Le, G. W. Oxidative stress induced by high-glucose diet in liver of C57BL/6J mice and its underlying mechanism. *Molecular Biology Reports* 2010; 37: 3833–9.

9. Hu, Y., Block, G., Norkus, E. P., Morrow, J. D., Dietrich, M. and Hudes, M. Relations of glycemic index and glycemic load with plasma oxidative stress markers. *The American Journal of Clinical Nutrition* 2006; 84: 70–6; quiz 266–7.

10. Liu, S. and Willett, W. C. Dietary glycemic load and atherothrombotic risk. *Current Atherosclerosis Reports* 2002; 4: 454–61.

11. Castro-Quezada, I., Sanchez-Villegas, A., Estruch, R., et al. A high dietary glycemic index increases total mortality in a Mediterranean population at high cardiovascular risk. *PloS One* 2014; 9: e107968.

12. Nielsen, F. H., Johnson, L. K. and Zeng, H. Magnesium supplementation improves indicators of low magnesium status and inflammatory stress in adults older than 51 years with poor quality sleep. *Magnesium Research: Official Organ of the International Society for the Development of Research on Magnesium* 2010; 23: 158–68.

13. Barbagallo, M. and Dominguez, L. J. Magnesium and aging. *Current Pharmaceutical Design* 2010; 16: 832–9.

14. La Vecchia, C. Tomatoes, lycopene intake, and digestive tract and female hormone-related neoplasms. *Experimental Biology and Medicine* 2002; 227: 860–3.

15. Wang, F., Dai, S., Wang, M. and Morrison, H. Erectile dysfunction and fruit/vegetable consumption among diabetic Canadian men. *Urology* 2013; 82: 1330–5.

16. Esposito, K., Giugliano, F., Di Palo, C., et al. Effect of lifestyle changes on erectile dysfunction in obese men: a randomized controlled trial. *JAMA* 2004; 291: 2978–84.

17. Esposito, K., Marfella, R., Ciotola, M., et al. Effect of a Mediterranean-style diet on endothelial dysfunction and markers of vascular inflammation in the metabolic syndrome: A randomized trial. *JAMA* 2004; 292: 1440–6.

18. Martinez-Lapiscina, E. H., Clavero, P., Toledo, E., et al. Mediterranean diet improves cognition: the PREDIMED-NAVARRA randomised trial. *Journal of 3, Neurosurgery, and Psychiatry* 2013; 84: 1318–25.

19. Gu, Y., Nieves, J. W, Stern, Y., Luchsinger, J. A. and Scarmeas, N. Food combination and Alzheimer disease risk: a protective diet. *Archives of Neurology* 2010; 67: 699–706.

20. Mosconi, L., Murray, J., Tsui, W. H., et al. Mediterranean diet and magnetic resonance imaging-assessed brain atrophy in cognitively normal individuals at risk for Alzheimer's disease. *The Journal of Prevention of Alzheimer's Disease* 2014; 1: 23–32.

21. Bjelakovic, G., Nikolova, D., Gluud, L. L., Simonetti, R. G. and Gluud, C. Mortality in randomized trials of antioxidant supplements for primary and secondary prevention: systematic review and meta-analysis. *JAMA* 2007; 297: 842–57.

CHAPTER 11

1. Rizzuto, D., Orsini, N., Qiu, C., Wang, H. X. and Fratiglioni, L. Lifestyle, social factors, and survival after age 75: population based study. *BMJ* 2012; 345: e5568.

2. Fratiglioni, L., Wang, H. X., Ericsson, K., Maytan, M., and Winblad, B. Influence of social network on occurrence of dementia: a community-based longitudinal study. *Lancet* 2000; 355: 1315–9.

3. Kaplan, R. M. and Kronick, R. G. Marital status and longevity in the United States population. *Journal of Epidemiology and Community Health* 2006; 60: 760–5.

4. Mainous, A. G, 3rd, Everett, C. J, Diaz, V. A., et al. Leukocyte telomere length and marital status among middle-aged adults. *Age and Ageing* 2011; 40: 73–8.

5. Zalli, A., Carvalho, L. A., Lin, J., et al. Shorter telomeres with high telomerase activity are associated with raised allostatic load and impoverished psychosocial resources. *Proceedings of the National Academy of Sciences of the United States of America* 2014; 111: 4519–24.

6. Tower, R. B., Kasl, S. V. and Darefsky, A. S. Types of marital closeness and mortality risk in older couples. *Psychosomatic Medicine* 2002; 64: 644–59.

7. Ballas, D. and Dorling, D. Measuring the impact of major life events upon happiness. *International Journal of Epidemiology* 2007; 36: 1244–52.

8. Pezzin, L. E., Pollak, R. A. and Schone, B. S. Complex families and late-life outcomes among elderly persons: Disability, institutionalization, and longevity. *Journal of Marriage and the Family* 2013; 75: 1084–97.

9. Hummer, R. A., Rogers, R. G., Nam, C. B. and Ellison, C. G. Religious involvement and U.S. adult mortality. *Demography* 1999; 36: 273–85.

10. Mitchell, B. D., Lee, W. J., Tolea, M. I., et al. Living the good life? Mortality and hospital utilization patterns in the Old Order Amish. *PloS One* 2012; 7: e51560.

11. Musick, M. A., House, J. S. and Williams, D. R. Attendance at religious services and mortality in a national sample. *Journal of Halth and Social Behavior* 2004; 45: 198–213.

12. Helm, H. M., Hays, J. C., Flint, E. P., Koenig, H. G. and Blazer, D. G. Does private religious activity prolong survival? A six-year follow-up study of 3,851 older

adults. *The Journals of Gerontology Series A, Biological Sciences and Medical Sciences* 2000; 55: M400–5.

13. Koenig, H. G., George, L. K. and Titus, P. Religion, spirituality, and health in medically ill hospitalized older patients. *Journal of the American Geriatrics Society* 2004; 52: 554–62.

14. Zeng, Y. and Shen, K. Resilience significantly contributes to exceptional longevity. *Current Gerontology and Geriatrics Research* 2010; 2010: 525693.

15. Kasen, S., Wickramaratne, P., Gameroff, M. J. and Weissman, M. M. Religiosity and resilience in persons at high risk for major depression. *Psychological Medicine* 2012; 42: 509–19.

16. Pargament, K. I., Koenig, H. G., Tarakeshwar, N. and Hahn, J. Religious struggle as a predictor of mortality among medically ill elderly patients: a 2-year longitudinal study. *Archives of Internal Medicine* 2001; 161: 1881–5.

17. Ford, E. S., Loucks, E. B. and Berkman, L. F. Social integration and concentrations of C-reactive protein among US adults. *Annals of Epidemiology* 2006; 16: 78–84.

18. Montross, L. P., Depp, C., Daly, J., et al. Correlates of self-rated successful aging among community-dwelling older adults. *The American Journal of Geriatric Psychiatry: Official Journal of the American Association for Geriatric Psychiatry* 2006; 14: 43–51.

19. Gleibs, I. H., Haslam, C., Jones, J. M., Alexander Haslam, S., McNeill, J. and Connolly, H. No country for old men? The role of a 'Gentlemen's Club' in promoting social engagement and psychological well-being in residential care. *Aging & Mental Health* 2011; 15: 456–66.

20. Kato, K., Zweig, R., Barzilai, N. and Atzmon, G. Positive attitude towards life and emotional expression as personality phenotypes for centenarians. *Aging* (Albany NY) 2012; 4: 359–67.

CHAPTER 12

1. Sutters, M. Systemic hypertension. In S. McPhee and M. A. Papdakis, eds, *Current Medical Diagnosis and Treatment*. New York McGraw Hill Medical, 2011.

2. Elliott, W. J. Compliance—and improving it—in hypertension. *Management Care* 2003; 12: 56–61.

3. Nelson, L., Gard, P. and Tabet, N. Hypertension and inflammation in Alzheimer's disease: close partners in disease development and progression! *Journal of Alzheimer's disease: JAD* 2014; 41: 331–43.

4. Prior, I. A., Evans, J. G., Harvey, H. P., Davidson, F. and Lindsey, M. Sodium intake and blood pressure in two Polynesian populations. *New England Journal of Medicine* 1968; 279: 515–20.

5. Coxson, P. G., Cook, N. R., Joffres, M., et al. Mortality benefits from US population-wide reduction in sodium consumption: projections from 3 modeling approaches. *Hypertension* 2013; 61: 564–70.

CHAPTER 13

1. Gilbert, D. *Stumbling on Happiness*. New York: Vintage Books, 2006.

2. Steptoe, A., Deaton, A. and Stone, A. A. Subjective wellbeing, health, and ageing. *Lancet* 2015; 385: 640–8.

3. Lawrence, E. M., Rogers, R. G., and Wadsworth, T. Happiness and longevity in the United States. *Social Science & Medicine* 2015; 45: 115–19,.

4. Kok, B. E., Coffey, K. A., Cohn, M. A., et al. How positive emotions build physical health: perceived positive social connections account for the upward spiral between positive emotions and vagal tone. *Psychological Science* 2013; 24: 1123–32.

5. Bernard, M., Braunschweig, G., Fegg, M. J. and Borasio, G. D. Meaning in life and perceived quality of life in Switzerland: results of a representative survey in the German, French and Italian regions. *Health and Quality of Life Outcomes* 2015; 13: 160.

6. Parker, S. J., Strath, S. J. and Swartz, A. M. Physical activity measurement in older adults: relationships with mental health. *Journal of Aging Physical Act* 2008; 16: 369–80.

7. Ali, A., Ambler, G., Strydom, A., et al. The relationship between happiness and intelligent quotient: the contribution of socio-economic and clinical factors. *Psychological Medicine* 2012; 43: 1303–12.

8. Kahneman, D., Krueger, A. B., Schkade, D., Schwarz, N. and Stone, A. A. Would you be happier if you were richer? A focusing illusion. *Science* 2006; 312: 1908–10.

9. Brickman, P., Coates, D. and Janoff-Bulman, R. Lottery winners and accident victims: is happiness relative? *Journal of Personality and Social Psychology* 1978; 36: 917–27.

10. Boyce, C. J., Brown, G. D. and Moore, S. C. Money and happiness: rank of income, not income, affects life satisfaction. *Psychological science* 2010; 21: 471–5.

11. Berthold, A. and Ruch, W. Satisfaction with life and character strengths of non-religious and religious people: it's practicing one's religion that makes the difference. *Frontiers in Psychology* 2014; 5: 876.

12. Stavrova, O., Fetchenhauer, D. and Schlosser, T. Why are religious people happy? The effect of the social norm of religiosity across countries. *Social Science Research* 2013; 42: 90–105.

13. Kasen, S., Wickramaratne, P., Gameroff, M. J. and Weissman, M. M. Religiosity and resilience in persons at high risk for major depression. *Psychological Medicine* 2012; 42: 509–19.

14. List of wars by death toll. In: https://en.wikipedia.org/wiki/List_of_wars_by_death_toll: wikipedia, 2015.

15. Lewis, M. B. and Bowler, P. J. Botulinum toxin cosmetic therapy correlates with a more positive mood. *Journal of Cosmetic Dermatology* 2009; 8: 24–6.

CHAPTER 14

1. Palfrey, S. Daring to practice low-cost medicine in a high-tech era. *The New England Journal of Medicine* 2011; 364: e21.
2. Zhi, M., Ding, E. L., Theisen-Toupal, J., Whelan, J., and Arnaout, R. The landscape of inappropriate laboratory testing: a 15-year meta-analysis. *PloS ONE* 2013; 8: e78962.
3. Ubel, P. A., Abernethy, A. P., and Zafar, S. Y. Full disclosure—out-of-pocket costs as side effects. *The New England Journal of Medicine* 2013; 369: 1484–6.

CHAPTER 15

1. Mukhopadhyay, D., and Mohanaruban, K. Iron deficiency anaemia in older people: investigation, management and treatment. *Age and Ageing* 2002; 31: 87–91.
2. Parmley, W. W. Prevalence and clinical significance of silent myocardial ischemia. *Circulation* 1989; 80: IV68–73.

CHAPTER 16

1. Simon, M. Timing when to take your daily medications. In: *AARP Bulletin*, 2013. http://www.aarp.org/health/drugs-supplements/info-12-2013/timing-of-daily-medications-key.html.
2. Schiele, J. T., Schneider, H., Quinzler, R., Reich, G., and Haefeli, W. E. Two techniques to make swallowing pills easier. *Annals of Family Medicine* 2014; 12: 550–2.
3. Ibid.
4. Marengoni, A., Pasina, L., Concoreggi, C., et al. Understanding adverse drug reactions in older adults through drug-drug interactions. *European Journal of Internal Medicine* 2014; 25: 843–6.
5. Franceschi, M., Scarcelli, C., Niro, V., et al. Prevalence, clinical features and avoidability of adverse drug reactions as cause of admission to a geriatric unit: a prospective study of 1756 patients. *Drug Safety: An International Journal of Medical Toxicology and Drug Experience* 2008; 31: 545–56.
6. Scott, I. A., Anderson, K., Freeman, C. R., and Stowasser, D. A. First do no harm: a real need to deprescribe in older patients. *The Medical Journal of Australia* 2014; 201: 390–2.
7. Green, J. L., Hawley, J. N., and Rask, K. J. Is the number of prescribing physicians an independent risk factor for adverse drug events in an elderly outpatient population? *The American Journal of Geriatric Pharmacotherapy* 2007; 5: 31–9.

8. Bonten, T. N., Saris, A., van Oostrom, M. J., et al. Effect of aspirin intake at bedtime versus on awakening on circadian rhythm of platelet reactivity. A randomised cross-over trial. *Thrombosis and Haemostasis* 2014; 112: 1209–18.

9. Suarez-Barrientos, A., Lopez-Romero, P., Vivas, D., et al. Circadian variations of infarct size in acute myocardial infarction. *Heart* 2011; 97: 970–6.

10. Huangfu, W., Duan, P., Xiang, D., and Gao, R. Administration time-dependent effects of combination therapy on ambulatory blood pressure in hypertensive subjects. *International Journal of Clinical and Experimental Medicine* 2015; 8: 19156–61.

11. Hermida, R. C., Ayala, D. E., Mojon, A., and Fernandez, J. R. Bedtime dosing of antihypertensive medications reduces cardiovascular risk in CKD. *Journal of the American Society of Nephrology: JASN* 2011; 22: 2313–21.

12. Bailey, D. G. Grapefruit-medication interactions. *CMAJ: Canadian Medical Association Journal = Journal de l'Association medicale canadienne* 2013; 185: 507–8.

13. Davit, B. M., Nwakama, P. E., Buehler, G. J., et al. Comparing generic and innovator drugs: a review of 12 years of bioequivalence data from the United States Food and Drug Administration. *The Annals of Pharmacotherapy* 2009; 43: 1583–97.

14. Kesselheim, A. S., Misono, A. S., Lee, J. L., et al. Clinical equivalence of generic and brand-name drugs used in cardiovascular disease: a systematic review and meta-analysis. *JAMA* 2008; 300: 2514–26.

15. Drug Expiration Dates—Do They Mean Anything? In: Harvard Health Publications, 2003. http://www.health.harvard.edu/fhg/updates/update1103a.shtml.

16. Lyon, R. C., Taylor, J. S., Porter, D. A., Prasanna, H. R., and Hussain, A. S. Stability profiles of drug products extended beyond labeled expiration dates. *Journal of Pharmaceutical Sciences* 2006; 95: 1549–60.

17. Cantrell, L., Suchard, J. R., Wu, A., and Gerona, R. R. Stability of active ingredients in long-expired prescription medications. *Archives of Internal Medicine* 2012; 172: 1685–7.

18. Pierson, J. C. Let's put an expiration date on the current approach to drug expiration dates. *Journal of the American Academy of Dermatology* 2014; 71: 193–4.

CHAPTER 17

1. Schnabel, K., Binting, S., Witt, C. M. and Teut, M. Use of complementary and alternative medicine by older adults—a cross-sectional survey. *BMC Geriatrics* 2014; 14: 38.

2. Kofoed, C. L., Christensen, J., Dragsted, L. O., Tjonneland, A. and Roswall N. Determinants of dietary supplement use—healthy individuals use dietary supplements. *The British Journal of Nutrition* 2015: 1–8.

3. van Rossem, K. and Lowe, J. A. A Phase 1, randomized, open-label crossover study to evaluate the safety and pharmacokinetics of 400 mg albaconazole administered to healthy participants as a tablet formulation versus a capsule formulation. *Clinical Pharmacology:Advances and Applications* 2013; 5: 23–31.

4. NIH. Supplements for Weight Loss Fact Sheet for Health Professionals. In: http://ods.od.nih.gov/factsheets/WeightLoss-HealthProfessional/Dietary NIH: Office of dietary supplements, 2015.

5. Dietary Supplements. In: http://www.fda.gov/Food/DietarySupplements/: FDA, 2015.

6. Zhou, S., Chan, E., Pan, S. Q., Huang, M. and Lee, E. J. Pharmacokinetic interactions of drugs with St John's wort. *Journal of Psychopharmacology* 2004; 18: 262–76.

7. The dangers of dietary and nutritional supplements investigated. In: What you don't know about these 12 ingredients could hurt you, http://www.consumerreports. org/cro/2012/05/dangerous-supplements/index.htm: Consumer Reports, 2010.

8. Conner, E. M. and Grisham, M. B. Inflammation, free radicals, and antioxidants. *Nutrition* 1996; 12: 274–7.

9. Bjelakovic, G., Nikolova, D., Gluud, L. L., Simonetti, R. G. and Gluud, C. Mortality in randomized trials of antioxidant supplements for primary and secondary prevention: systematic review and meta-analysis. *JAMA* 2007; 297: 842–57.

10. Soare, A., Weiss, E. P., Holloszy, J. O. and Fontana, L. Multiple dietary supplements do not affect metabolic and cardio-vascular health. *Aging* (Albany NY) 2014; 6: 149–57.

11. Guigoz, Y. and Vellas, B. J. Malnutrition in the elderly: the Mini Nutritional Assessment (MNA). *Therapeutische Umschau Revue therapeutique* 1997; 54: 345–50.

12. Annweiler, C., Kabeshova, A., Legeay, M., Fantino, B. and Beauchet, O. Derivation and validation of a clinical diagnostic tool for the identification of older community-dwellers with hypovitaminosis D. *Journal of the American Medical Directors Association* 2015; 16: 536.

13. Lindenbaum, J., Rosenberg, I. H., Wilson, P. W., Stabler, S. P. and Allen, R. H. Prevalence of cobalamin deficiency in the Framingham elderly population. *The American Journal of Clinical Nutrition* 1994; 60: 2–11

14. Petridou, E. T., Kousoulis, A. A., Michelakos, T., et al. Folate and B12 serum levels in association with depression in the aged: a systematic review and meta-analysis. *Aging & Mental Health* 2015; 20: 965–78.

15. Mulholland, P. J., Self, R. L., Stepanyan, T. D., Little, H. J., Littleton, J. M. and Prendergast, M. A. Thiamine deficiency in the pathogenesis of chronic ethanol-associated cerebellar damage in vitro. *Neuroscience* 2005; 135: 1129–39.

16. Prior, I. A., Evans, J. G., Harvey, H. P., Davidson, F. and Lindsey, M. Sodium intake and blood pressure in two Polynesian populations. *The New England Journal of Medicine* 1968; 279: 515–20.

17. Yang, Q., Liu, T., Kuklina, E. V., et al. Sodium and potassium intake and mortality among US adults: prospective data from the Third National Health and Nutrition Examination Survey. *Archives of Internal Medicine* 2011; 171: 1183–91.

18. Nielsen, F. H., Johnson, L. K. and Zeng, H. Magnesium supplementation improves indicators of low magnesium status and inflammatory stress in adults older than 51 years with poor quality sleep. *Magnesium Research: Official Organ of the*

International Society for the Development of Research on Magnesium 2010; 23: 158–68.

19. Wark, P. A., Lau, R., Norat, T. and Kampman, E. Magnesium intake and colorectal tumor risk: a case-control study and meta-analysis. *The American Journal of Clinical Nutrition* 2012; 96: 622–36.

20. Clarke, B. L., Ebeling, P. R., Jones, J. D., et al. Predictors of bone mineral density in aging healthy men varies by skeletal site. *Calcified Tissue International* 2002; 70: 137–45.

21. Samaras, N., Papadopoulou, M. A., Samaras, D. and Ongaro, F. Off-label use of hormones as an antiaging strategy: a review. *Clinical Interventions in Aging* 2014; 9: 1175–86.

CHAPTER 18

1. Earle, C. C., Neville, B. A., Landrum, M. B., Ayanian, J. Z., Block, S. D. and Weeks, J. C. Trends in the aggressiveness of cancer care near the end of life. *Journal of Clinical Oncology* 2004; 22: 315–21.

2. Gallo, J. J., Straton, J. B., Klag, M. J., et al. Life-sustaining treatments: what do physicians want and do they express their wishes to others? *Journal of the American Geriatrics Society* 2003; 51: 961–9.

3. Jones, J. W. and McCullough, L. B. Futility and surgical intervention. *Journal of Vascular Surgery* 2002; 35: 1305.

Index

About the Author

James W. Jones is well-qualified on matters concerning successful aging. He attended Tulane Medical School on scholarship and became an honor society student. His education continued with fellowships at the Mayo and Ochsner Clinics and residency at Tulane. Next, he earned a PhD in cell biology and studied how cancer cells multiply and how heart muscle energizes. He was a faculty member at Tulane and then the Baylor College of Medicine under Dr. Michael DeBakey during the golden age of cardiovascular surgery. He moved on to become distinguished professor and Hugh Stephenson Chair of Surgery at the University of Missouri. During this time he earned a Master of Health Administration, which was his last degree. During his career, he performed over 12,000 procedures and published three books and over 400 other publications. He has many awards for research, education, and medical leadership.